Orlando Castejón

Basic and Clinical Neuroscience Researcher Profile

Orlando Castejón

Basic and Clinical Neuroscience Researcher Profile

Histochemical Study of Proteoglycans and Childhood Malnutrition

ScienciaScripts

Imprint

Cover image: www.ingimage.com

This book is a translation from the original published under ISBN 978-613-9-40446-9.

Publisher:
Sciencia Scripts
is a trademark of
Dodo Books Indian Ocean Ltd. and OmniScriptum S.R.L publishing group

120 High Road, East Finchley, London, N2 9ED, United Kingdom
Str. Armeneasca 28/1, office 1, Chisinau MD-2012, Republic of Moldova, Europe
Printed at: see last page
ISBN: 978-620-8-05353-6

DR. HAYDÉE VILORIA DE CASTEJÓN. PROFILE OF A RESEARCHER IN BIOMEDICINE

ORLANDO J. CASTEJÓN

PREFACE

This academic monograph of Dr. Haydée Viloria de Castejón contains her family group, academic organisation, research activities, training of technical and scientific staff, participation in the organisation of research units, centres and institutes and research councils, organisation of national and international congresses, academic trips, participation in basic and clinical neuroscience research. It also includes the opinion of his relatives and professionals who contributed to and admire his scientific work.

DEDICATION

To his brothers:

Mará Elena Viloria de Alvarado, Nelly Viloria Ocando, Luis Viloria, Jesús Viloria, Gladys Viloria Ocando, Elsa Viloria de Silva, Yolanda Viloria de Litwinenko.

To his colleagues: Jorimar Leal, Pablo Ortega, María Elena Viloria de Alvarado.

To her friends Thais Urdaneta de Prado and Dora Freites.

CONTENT

CHAPTER I

THE VILORIA FAMILY OCANDO

Dr. Haydée Viloria Ocando's parents lived in Maracaibo. Venezuela (1961)

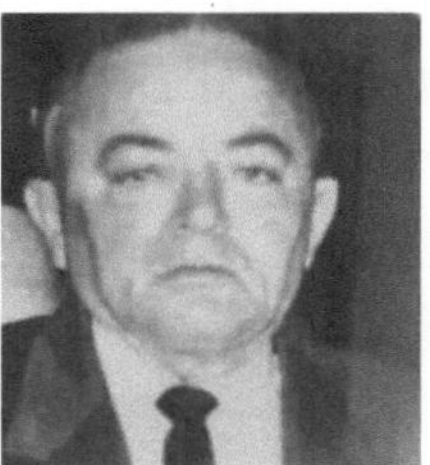

Mr. Luis

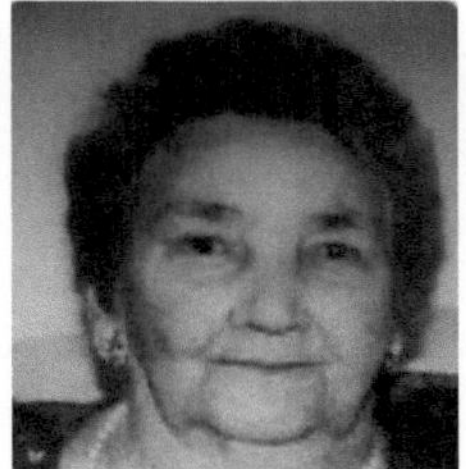

ViloriaMrs Julia Ocando de Viloria

The Viloria Ocando Family consisted of their children Haydée Viloria Ocando, Luis Viloria Ocando, Nelly Viloria Ocando, Mario Viloria Ocando, Maria Elena Viloria Ocando, Yolanda Viloria Ocando, Mario Viloria Ocando, Jesus Viloria Ocando 1and Luis Ramón Viloria.

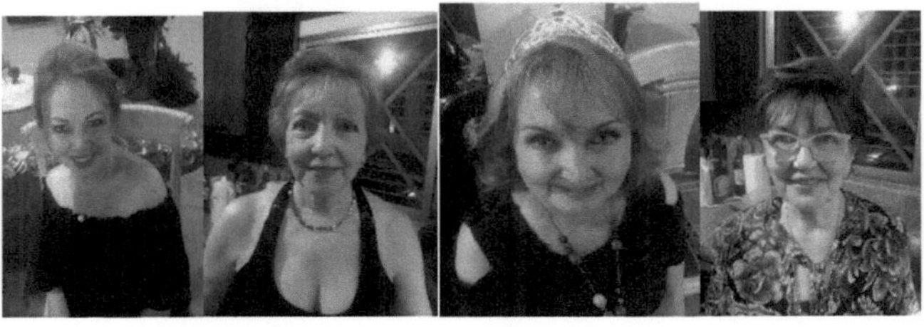

CHAPTER II

PRIMARY, SECONDARY AND UNIVERSITY EDUCATION

Haydée Viloria Ocando attended primary and secondary school at the Colegio Nuestra Señora del Pilar between 1946 and 1956.

He entered the Faculty of Medicine at the University of Zulia in 1956 and obtained his degree as a Surgeon in 1961.

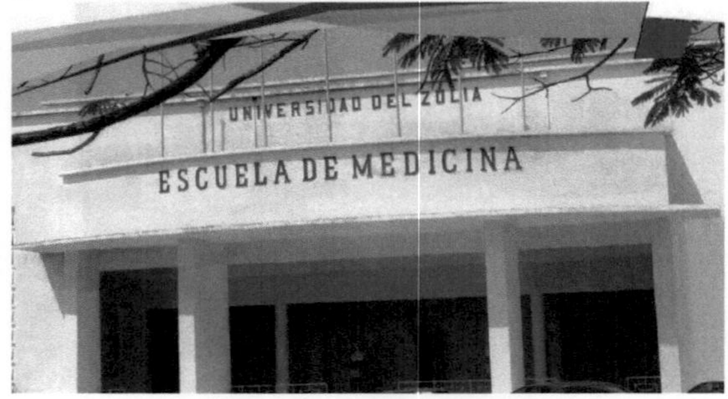

Graduation as Medical Surgeon (1962).

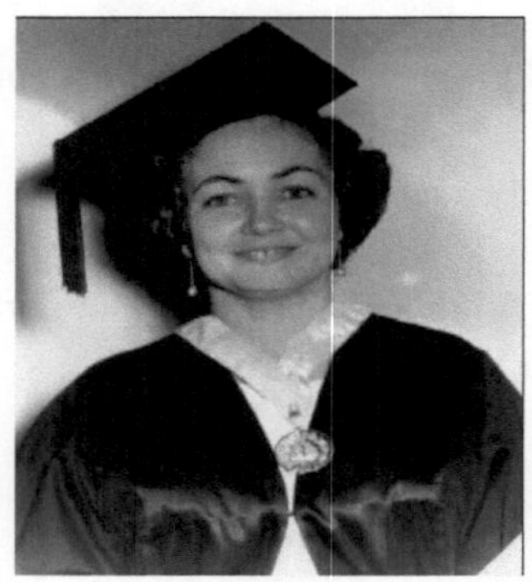

CHAPTER III

HISTOLOGY AND EMBRYOLOGY CHAIR TRAINER

In 1964, after her first year of medical school, she was appointed trainee in the Histology and Embryology Laboratory of the Faculty of Medicine under the direction of Dr. Franz Wenger, a renowned German pathologist.

Start in biomedical research

In 1958, Dr. Américo Negrette, Professor of Neurological Semiology at the Central Hospital Dr. Urquinaona, initiated her in the principles of medical research together with a group of medical students, including Elena and Slavia Ryder, Dora Freites, Jesús Rubio, Orlando Castejón and Professors Gabriel Díaz Sulbaran and Heberto Quintana Márquez. It was an emotional and happy start to microscopic research. Dr. Negrette, as we called him familiarly, a particularly charismatic Professor, remarkable writer and delicate painter, had distinguished himself for his clinical studies in Venezuelan Equine Encephalitis and in Hutington's Korea 2 during his tenure as a rural doctor in San Francisco, Maracaibo, Zulia State, Zulia State, he had the original idea, the gift of persuasion and the subtle conviction to bring together in those years, 1958 and 1959, a group of students, who today can be considered the forerunners of biomedical research in the Faculty of Medicine of the University of Zulia.

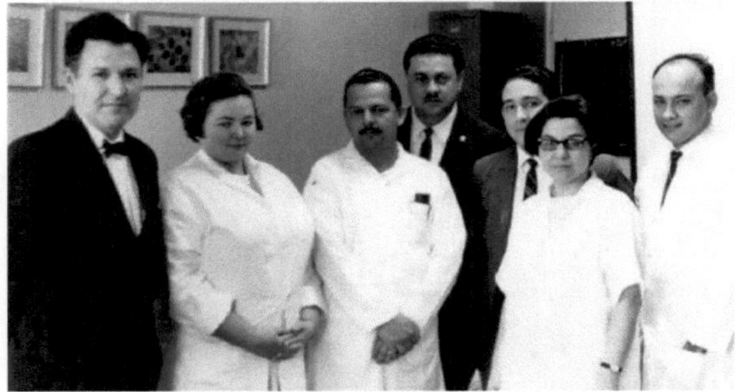

Dr Castejón with Dr Américo Negrette, Drs Castejón, Tyder, Soto and national guests.

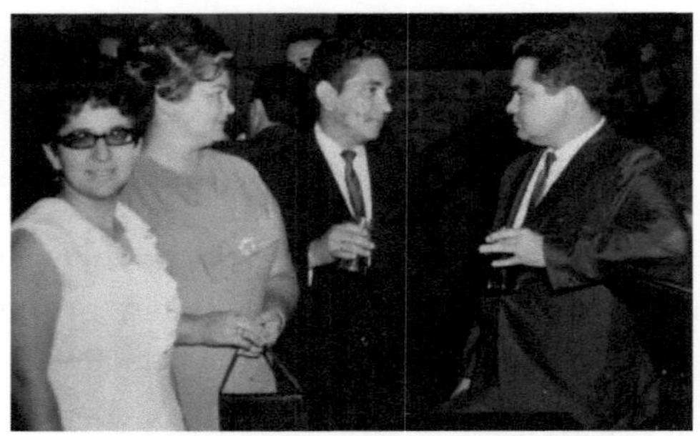

Drs. Castejón accompanied by Drs. Elena Ryder and Luis Viloria Ocando.

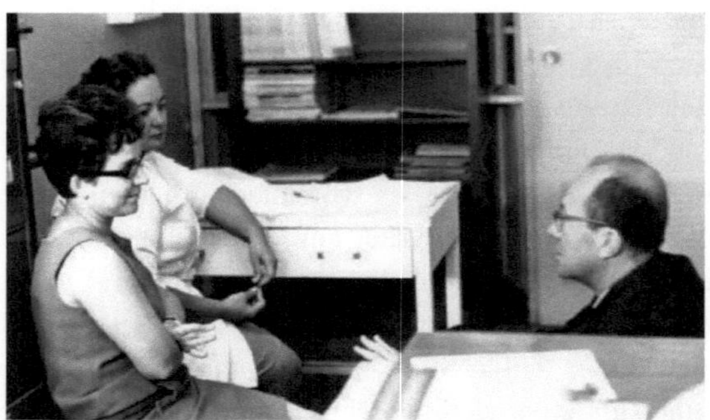

Dr. Castejón and Elena vonersando with Dr. Guillermo Whitembury, IVIC researcher and specialist in renal research (1962).

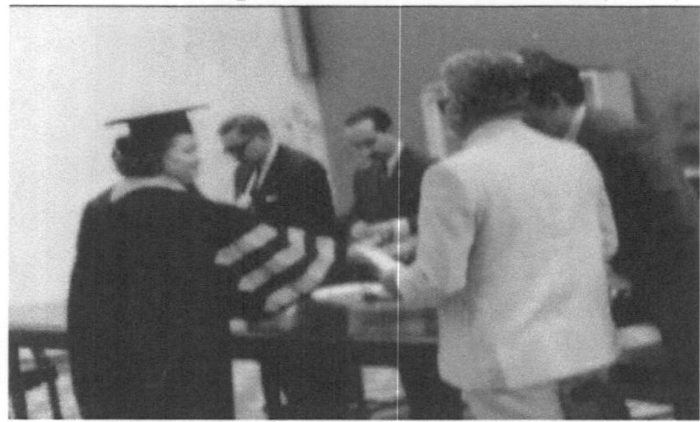

Receiving his degree of Doctor of Medical Sciences from the University Authorities Dr José Manuel Delgado Ocando, Rector and Regulo Pachano Añez (Academic Vice-Rector) (1970).

Showing his histochemical findings at the Biological Research Unit (1973).

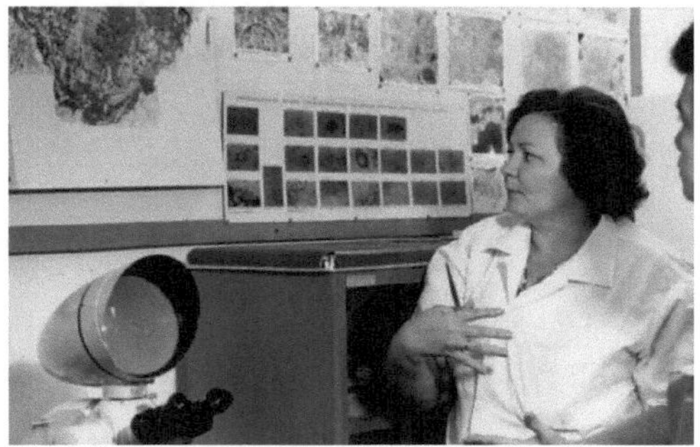

Receiving the Jesús Enrique Lossada Order imposed by the Rector of LUZ, Ing. José Ferrer (1989).

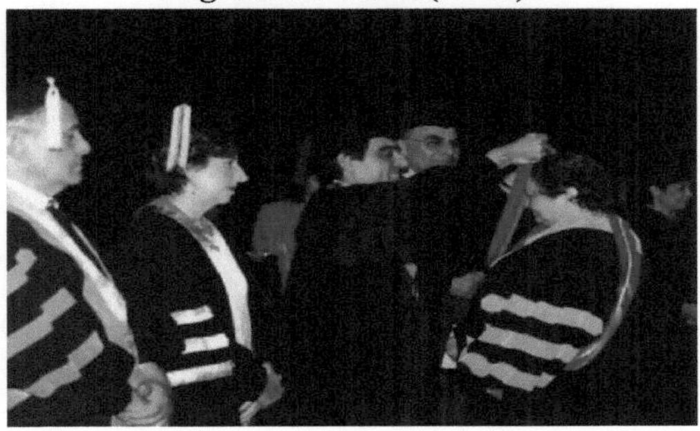

CHAPTER IV

POSTGRADUATE STUDIES AT THE INSTITUTO VENEZOLANO DE INVESTIGACIONES CIENTÍFICA (IVIC). ALTOS DE PIPE. MIRANDA STATE

To Dr. Marcel Roche and his always distinguished friendship and solidarity with Dr. Américo Negrette we owe this exceptional opportunity for scientific training of young researchers in the country, especially for the Clinical Research Institute of the Faculty of Medicine of the University of Zulia.

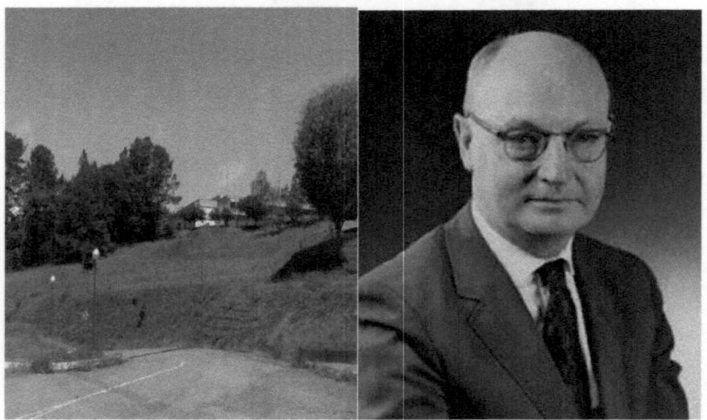

Photo IVIC. Altos de Pipe. Miranda State, Dr. Marcel Roche, Director of IVIC.

Dr Marcel Roche was a leading researcher in infantile parasitosis, coming from the Roche Foundation, an institution that housed the most distinguished researchers of the time.

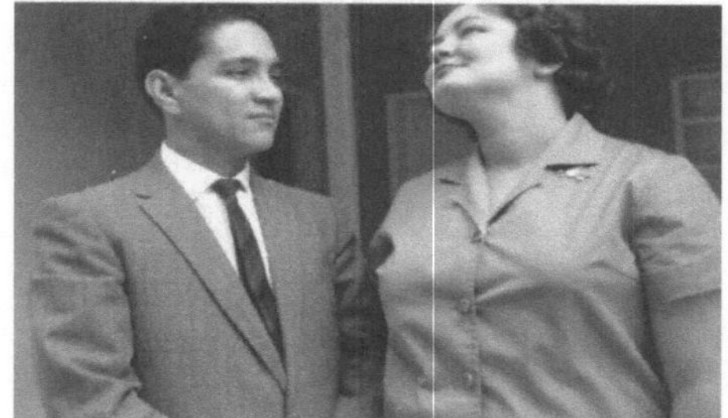

Drs. Haydée Viloria de Castejón and Orlando Castejón, IVIC Graduate Students (1963)

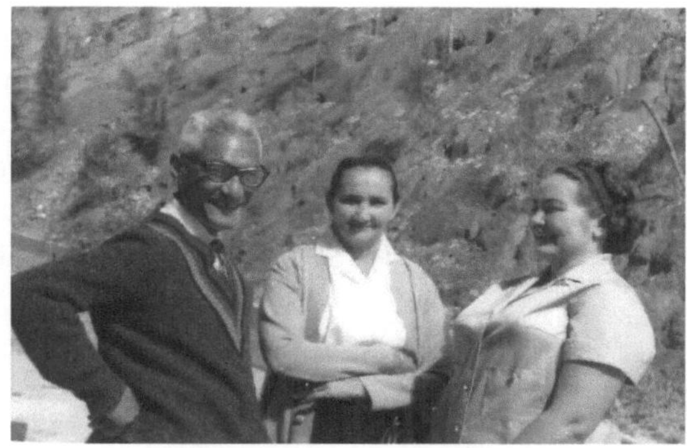

Our companions in House 4 of the IVIC, my father Clemente Castejón, Doña Julia Viloria Ocando and Haydée Viloria Ocando, from whom we received company and moral support in our postgraduate studies, for the first time outside Maracaibo (1963).

Dr. Haydée Viloria de Castejón and her postgraduate training at the Laboratory of Experimental Pathology directed by Dr. Luis Carbonell (1975) during 1962 and 1963.

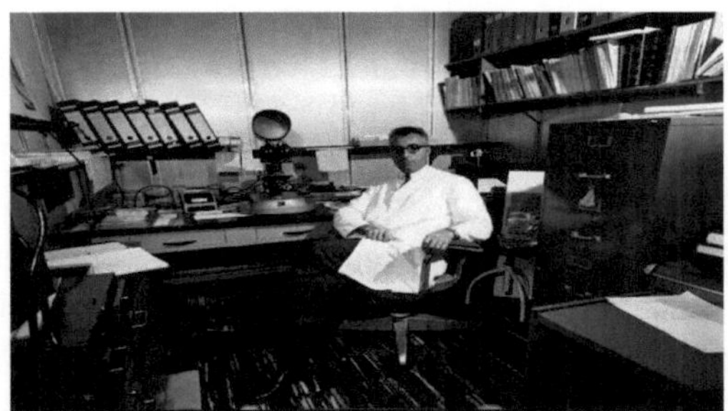

Dr. Luis Carbonell, Head of the Experimental Pathology Laboratory at IVIC (1972).

Postgraduate Fellowship in Neuroscience, Histochemistry and Cytochemistry at the University of California. Los Angeles (UCLA).

In January 1962, I travelled with my wife Dr. Haydee Vitoria de Castejón and my first daughter Orlhay Beatriz, as postgraduate scholarship holders from IVIC and the University of Zulia to continue our studies at the University of

California as Fellows in Electron Microscopy, Histochemistry and Cytochemistry. We had travelled to Los Angeles in the company of Evangela Castejón, our first cousin and long-time companion, who was constantly and devotedly taking care of Orlhay Beatriz. In Los Angeles we arrived at my sister Nelly's house in Hawthorne, and stayed there for several months until we moved to a flat in Culver City, an area closer to the University of California at Los Angeles (UCLA).

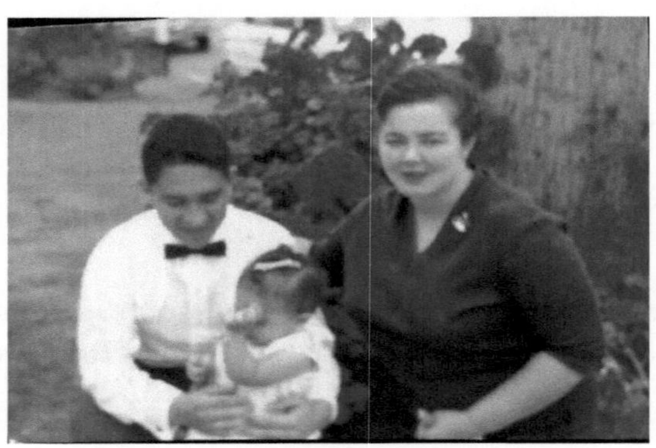

Drs. Castejón and their little daughter Orlhay Beatriz in Los Angeles (1964).

In February 1964, we formally began our studies of electron microscopy, cell biology and ultrastructure of the vertebrate retina at the Department of Zoology of the University of California Los Angeles (UCLA), now the Institute of Molecular Biology, Los Angeles (UCLA), under the direction of Professor Fritiof Sjostrand, a distinguished researcher from the Karolinska Institute in Stockholm, and a pioneer, together with Humberto Fernández Morán, of transmission electron microscopy in the world. Professor Sjostrand was accompanied by a group of researchers, including Ulf Karlsson, Lars Elfvin and Birguita Peterson, with whom she worked directly on intravascular perfusion fixation of the brain of rhesus monkeys to study the retina. Dr. Castejón was then placed in Dr. Jan Brown's Histochemistry Laboratory at the Brain Research Institute of the University of California.

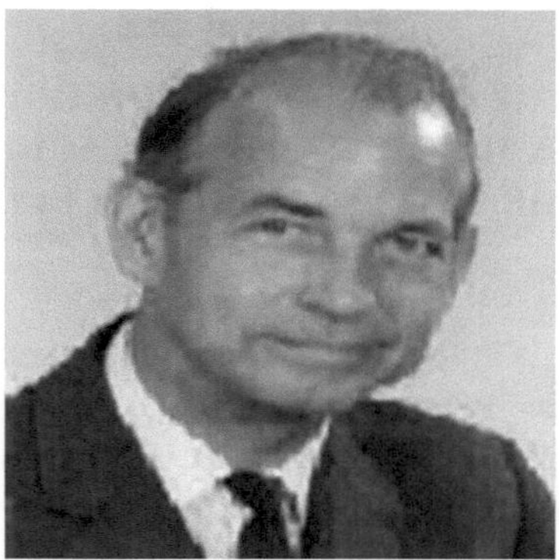

Professor Fritiof Sjöstrand, Research Fellow at the Karolinska Institute in Stockholm and Research Fellow in the Department of Zoology at the University of California.

CHAPTER V

HIS RETURN TO VENEZUELA AND HIS INCORPORATION TO THE CLINICAL RESEARCH CENTRE OF THE FACULTY OF MEDICINE OF THE UNIVERSITY OF ZULIA (1964)

We returned to Venezuela at the end of 1963 to reintegrate and work as contract professors at the Clinical Research Centre directed by Dr. Américo Negrette. Under the deanship of Dr. Enrique Molina, a Siemens electron microscope had been acquired, and once it was installed in the basement of the University Hospital, we were asked to return to Maracaibo. It was really a very premature return, but we were responding to the request of Dr. Enrique Molina and Dr. Amétrico Negrette.This was the end of a period of academic training and we had to assume our contractual commitment to the University of Zulia. Professor Sjöstrand offered us to continue our work in his department, but we felt that our destiny was the Faculty of Medicine of the University of Zulia. We had learned from our daily reading of the monographs of Don Santiago Ramon y Cajal that the most important thing for a scientist was his patriotic spirit. Otherwise American life would not offer us the attraction and stability for our destiny. Dr. Américo Negrete was not only his teacher, but also our compadre, as he was the godfather together with his wife Beatriz of our daughter Orlhay Beatriz. Today I think that this decision to return to the country was the right one and that it allowed us to collaborate in the foundation of biomedical research at the University of Zulia, especially in the Faculty of Medicine. At the Clinical Research Centre, later transformed into the Clinical Research Institute, we set up a working team that cooperated with the rest of the Institute's members for eight years. In this institution, Dr. Haydée Viloria de Castejón founded the Histochemistry and Cytochemistry Section (1964) and began her work by training the Laboratory Technicians Digna Peña and Neila Bohórquez, and establishing her lines of research in the histochemical study of proteoglycans in the optical and electronic microscope of the mouse cerebellum.He made his first publications in the Revista Investigación Clínica, the Journal of the Research Institute founded by Dr. Americo Negrette. In this Institution we had as co-workers Laboratorian Gabriel Sulbaran Solís, Internist Hernán Feréira, our colleagues from medical and postgraduate studies at IVIC, Dr. Elena and Slavia Ryder and Dr. Armando Soto Escalona.

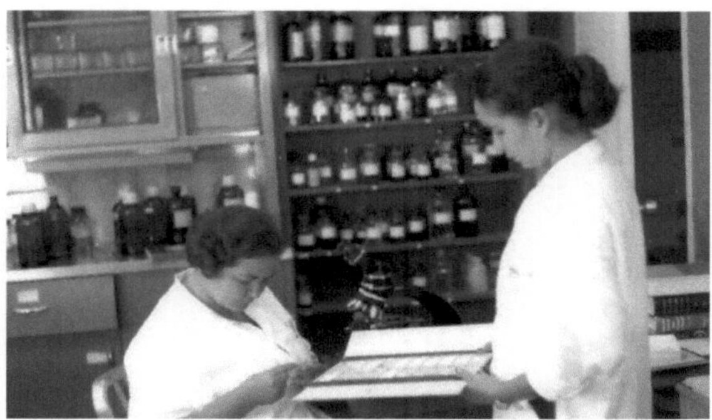

Dr. Haydée Viloria de Castejón and Digna de Bohórquez in the Histochemistry Laboratory at the Clinical Research Institute (1965). The Histochemistry technique Digna Bohórquez was trained by Dr. Castejón. She started her research at the Centro de Investigaciones Clínicas in Maracaibo. Venezuela located on the third floor of the University Hospital.

Dr. Américo Negrette Director of the Clinical Research Centre at the Hospital Universitario de Maracaibo (1965)

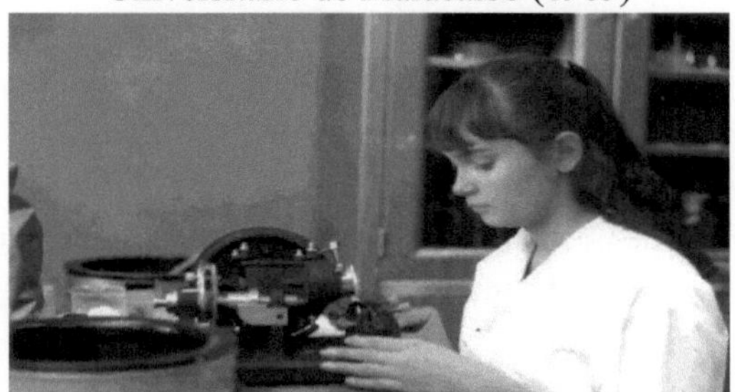

Neila Bohórquez. Histochemistry technique was trained to perform microtomy for thick paraffin sections of mouse cerebellum for staining with Alcian Blue.

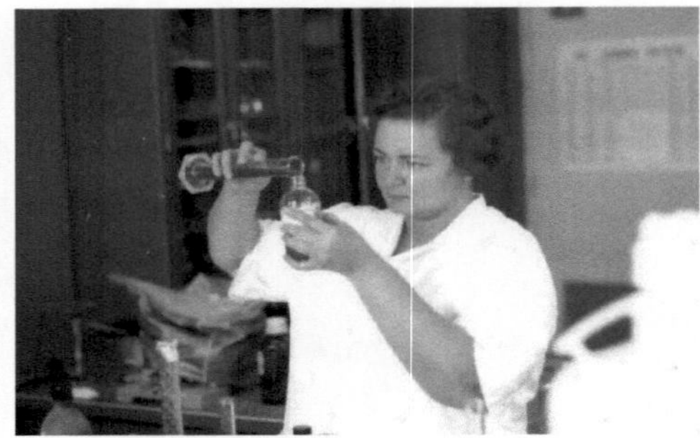

Dr. Haydée Viloria de Castejón in the Histochemistry Laboratory at the Clinical Research Institute preparing Alcian Blue stains for the determination of acid mucopolysaccharides in the mouse nervous system (1965).

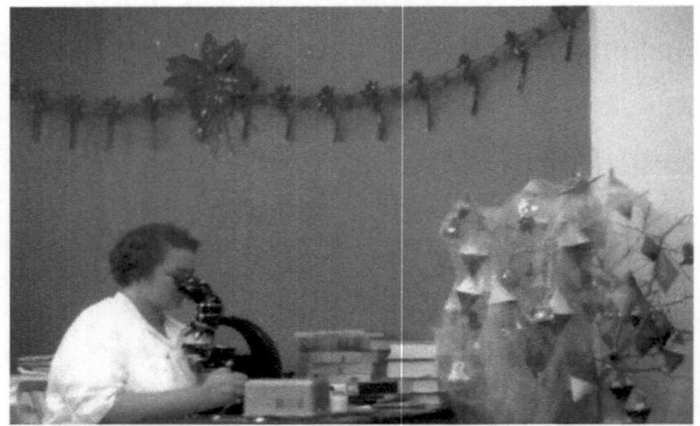

Dr. Haydée Viloria de Castejón looking at histochemical preparations of acid mucopolysaccharides in the mouse cerebellum under the light microscope.

We had entered the University of Zulia by competition as contract professors, and we remained in this situation for three years, until our entry as regular professors after a competitive examination.

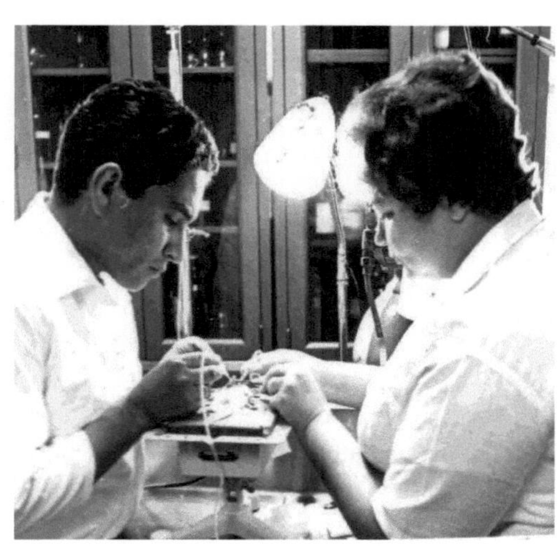

Drs Castejón performing intravascular perfusion of Swiss albino mouse brain with glutaraldehyde solution for transmission electron microscopy.

Monthly seminars on research programmes led by Dr. Américo Negrette were held at the Institute.

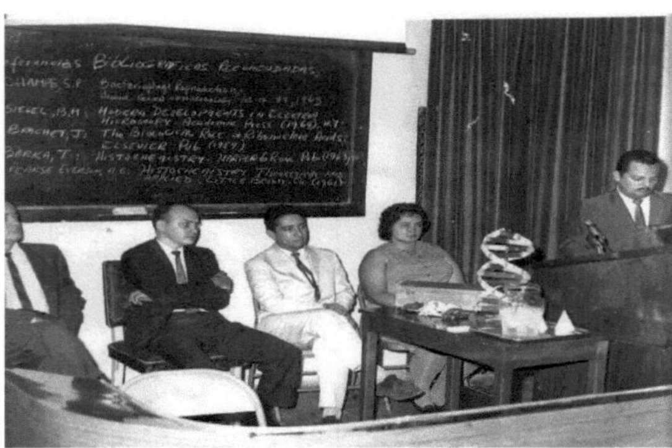

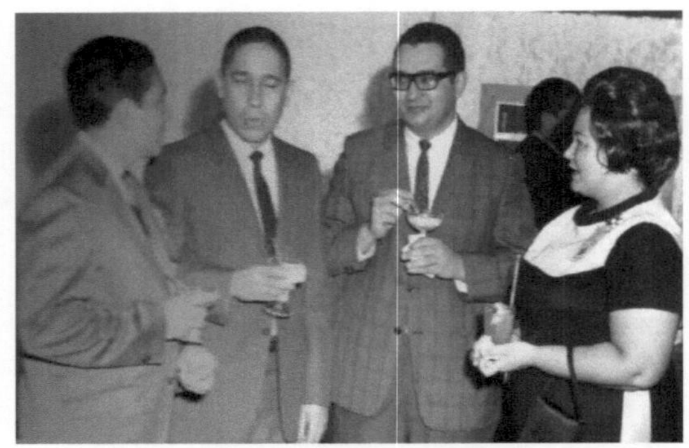

Drs. Castejón in conversation with Prof. Gilberto Olivares and Prof. José Ramón Guzmán attending the seminar.

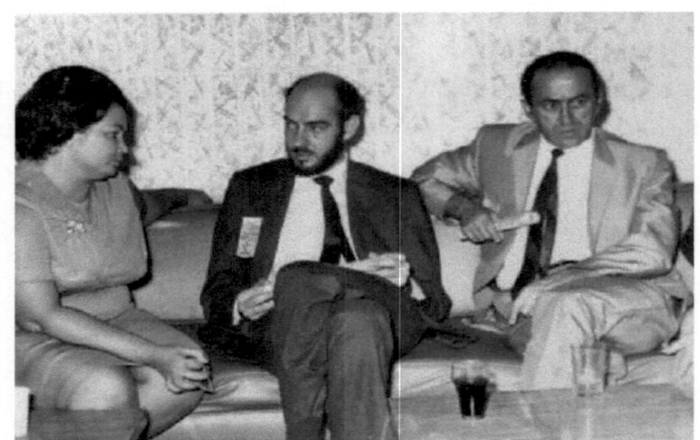

Dr. Castejón accompanied by Dr. Miguel Lauffer and Dr. Miguel Chuchani, prominent IVIC researchers (1967).

CHAPTER VI

THE CREATION OF THE BIOLOGICAL RESEARCH UNIT OF THE FACULTY OF MEDICINE OF THE UNIVERSITY OF ZULIA (1971)

The Biological Research Unit was approved by the Council of the Faculty of Medicine on 10 November 1971. Three research programmes were initiated, devoted to the study of proteoglycans in the central nervous system, microstructure and histochemistry of the vertebrate cerebellar cortex, and submicroscopic analysis of the pathological human cerebral cortex.

Our creation project contained the following objectives:

1) To carry out basic and applied research in the area of Biology and Experimental Medicine.
2) To promote and stimulate the development of scientific research in Basic Medical Sciences.
3) To project scientific research towards teaching by incorporating the principles and methodology of scientific research into the training of university students.

The Biological Research Unit started with two research sections: the Electron Microscopy Section and the Histochemistry Section, directed by Dr. Orlando J. Castejón and Dr. Haydée Viloria de Castejón, who acted as founding researchers. The following research programmes were established:

Section of Histochemistry and Cytochemistry.

Prof. in charge: Dr. Haydee Viloria de Castejón. Field of Research: Cell Biology, Histochemistry and Cytochemistry of Macromolecules.

Research Projects.

Acid mucopolysaccharides from nerve tissue:

1. Comparative study of acid mucopolysaccharides in the central nervous system of different vertebrates.
2. Electronohistochemical study of acid mucopolysaccharides in nervous tissue.
3. Acid mucopolysaccharides in the central nervous system of mice at different stages of brain development. Histochemical study.
4. Relationship between the acetylcholine system and acid mucopolysaccharides. Histochemical and electronomicroscopic study in the

mouse central nervous system.

The research programme directed by Dr. Haydée Viloria de Castejón on Histochemistry of Polysaccharides in the Nervous System initially produced 43 publications in the form of original articles, communications to congresses, and conferences published in international journals. This programme led to the discovery of new macromolecules within nerve cells, hyaluronic acid and chondroitin 4 and 6 sulphate, macromolecules traditionally conceptualised as constituents of extracellular spaces, which were found for the first time inside nerve cells. This finding was published in histochemical journals in Germany and the U.S.A. It was later confirmed by American and European researchers. In a book published in New York on Complex Carbohydrate Histochemistry by Richard Margolis (1980), the priority of the findings was given to Dr. Castejón and it is stated textually that the most extensive contribution to the study of these macromolecules in the nervous system was made by Dr. Viloria, citing more than 9 of her research works on this subject. Such The research was partially funded by CONICIT of the Republic of Venezuela and CONDES of the University of Zulia.

Drs. Castejón trained as teaching and research fellows Dr. María Elena Viloria, Dr. Consuelo Valero, María Palmar, and Alan Castellanos who later became researchers in the laboratory, and later directors of the Institute of Biological Research.

Dr. Haydée Viloria de Castejón and Dr. María Elena Viloria published an excellent monograph on Histochemical Techniques, with special emphasis on the demonstration of proteoglycans.

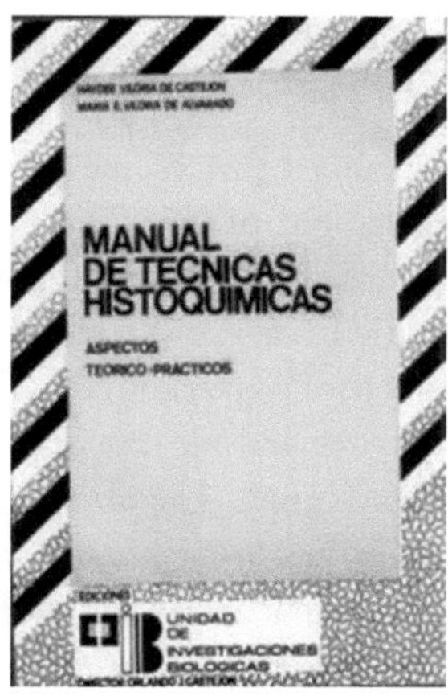

Contents Introduction
The Optical Microscope
Application of dyes in Histology and Histochemistry Chemical fixation of tissues for Histochemistry Freeze fixation of tissues

Lipids

Histochemistry of complex carbohydrates Histochemical demonstration of proteins Histochemistry of Nucleic Acids Principles of Enzymatic Histochemistry Preparation of buffer solutions Manufacturers of Histochemistry Equipment Specialist Histochemistry Journals Reference Texts Bibliographical references.

Incorporation of Technical Staff in the Histochemistry Laboratory

In this new institution we progressively incorporated, according to budget availability, the new technical personnel necessary to continue our research work, such as the Photographic Technician Nancy Rincón, the receptionist Beatriz Ocando, the Secretary of the Directorate Miriam Arenas, and the Lic. Josefina de Vivas for the Library of the Biological Research Unit, later converted into the Bibliographic Documentation Centre.

Transformation of the Biological Research Unit into the Biological Research Institute (1981).

In 1981 the Council of the Faculty of Medicine and the University Council of LUZ approved the transformation of the Biological Research Unit. The University of Zulia was awarded the title of Instituto de Investigaciones Biológicas, which was ratified in 1988 by the Consejo Nacional de Universidades (National Council of Universities). Obtaining the support of the University of Zulia was for Haydee and me one of the most important stimuli in the development of our academic career. The alma mater welcomed us back into its bosom and the postnubila phoebus of its emblem enlightened us forever. That is why we dedicated our lives to that University, which through its professors and authorities made possible the emergence of a new research unit in the Faculty of Medicine. We continued our lines of research and projects that we had started at the Clinical Research Institute, mainly devoted to the study of the microstructure and histochemistry of the cerebellar cortex of most vertebrates on the phylogenetic scale.

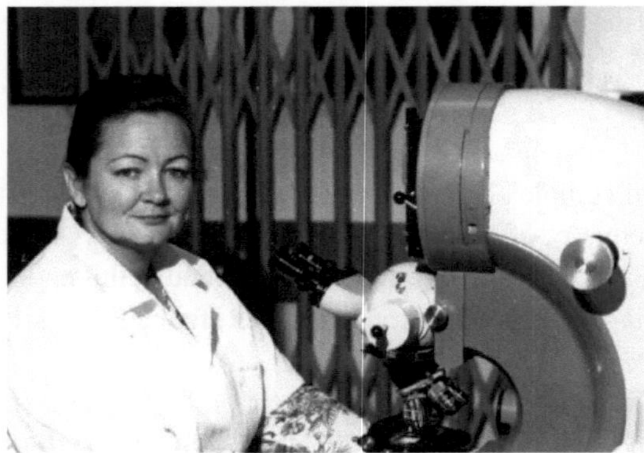

Dr. Viloria de Castejón with the Leitz photomicroscope to characterise proteoglycans in semi-thin sections embedded in plastic.

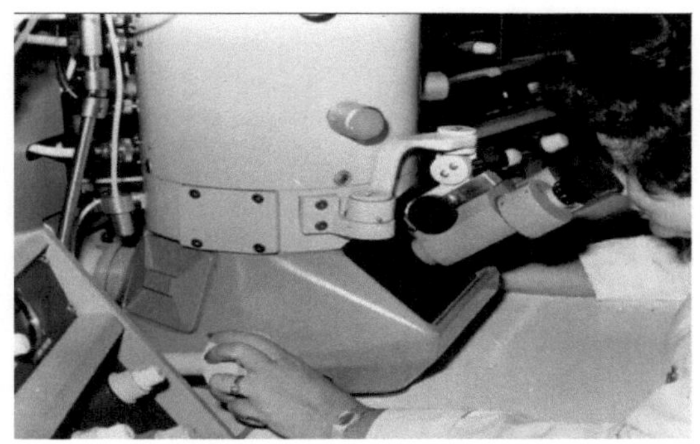

Dr. Viloria de Castejón observing ultra-thin sections of mouse cerebellum stained with the Gabould Method under the JEOL 100B electron microscope

Eminent Visitor: Dr. Eduardo de Robertis

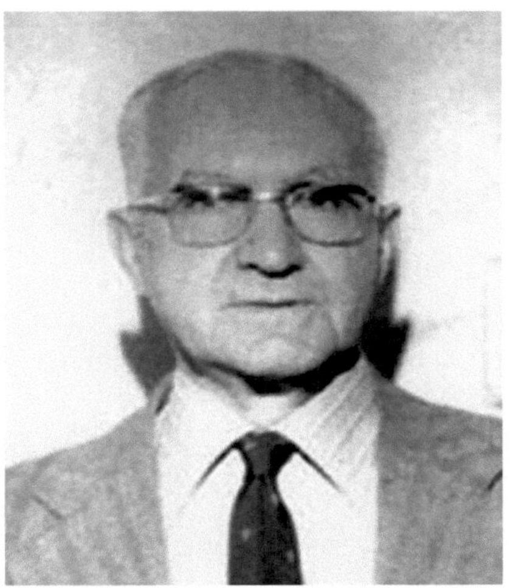

Dr. Eduardo De Robertis. Prominent Argentinean scientist. Director of the Institute of Cell Biology of the Faculty of Medicine of the University of Buenos Aires. Author together with Nowisnky and Saez of the book Cell Biology, official text used in the Faculties of Medicine of Latin American Universities.

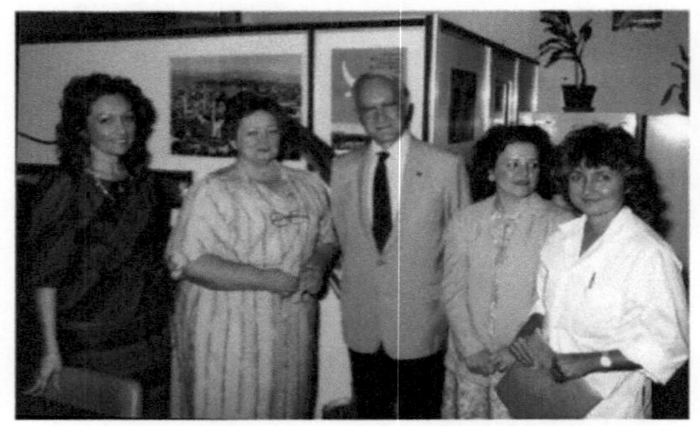

Dr Eduardo De Robertis. Visiting our Biological Research Institute with Dr Isabel Añez, Dr Haydeé Viloria de Castejón, Dr Clarisa Faria and Dr María Elena Viloria.

CHAPTER VII
PARTICIPATION OF DR. HAYDÉE VILORIA DE CASTEJÓN IN THE ORGANISATION OF NATIONAL AND INTERNATIONAL SCIENTIFIC SOCIETIES

The Foundation of the Zulia Chapter of the Venezuelan Association for the Advancement of Science.

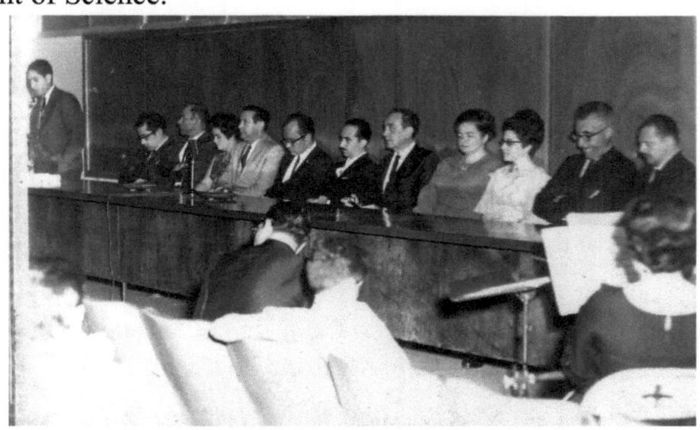

Members of the presidium at the installation of the Zuliano Chapter of ASOVAC. Distinguished from left to right are Drs. Américo Negrette, Luis Carbonell, Slavia Ryder, Haydée Viloria de Castejón, Bernardo Rodríguez D'Empaire, José Manuel Delgado Ocando, Jorge Villegas, Enrique Molina, Gloria Mercader de Villegas, Ernesto Medina and Raimundo Villegas.

Participation in the organisation of the First Latin American Congress on Electron Microscopy (ICLAME) in Maracaibo. Venezuela (1972)

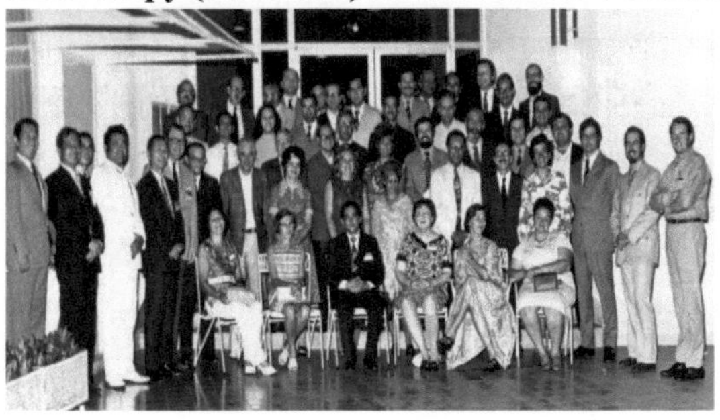

Participants of the I ICLAME. From left to right Drs. Stanley Barnett, Orlando Castejón, Haydée Castejón, Arnold Seligman, Antonio Serrano, and Pinto Da Silva.

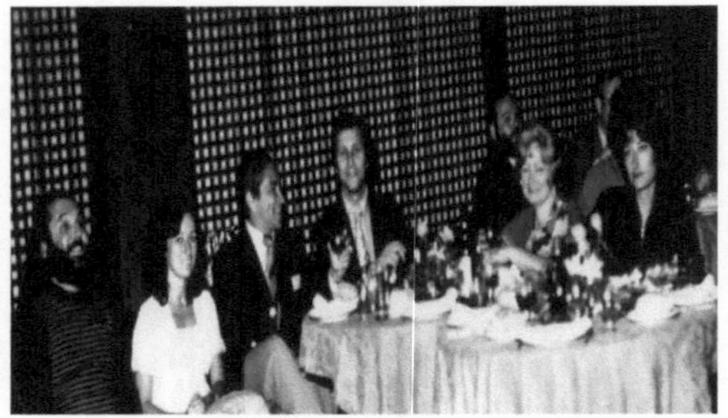

Participants of the 1st ICLAME. Among others, from left to right

José Antonio Serrano (ULA), Orlando Castejón (LUZ), Jaime Pereda Tapiol (Chile) and Haydée Viloria de Castejón.

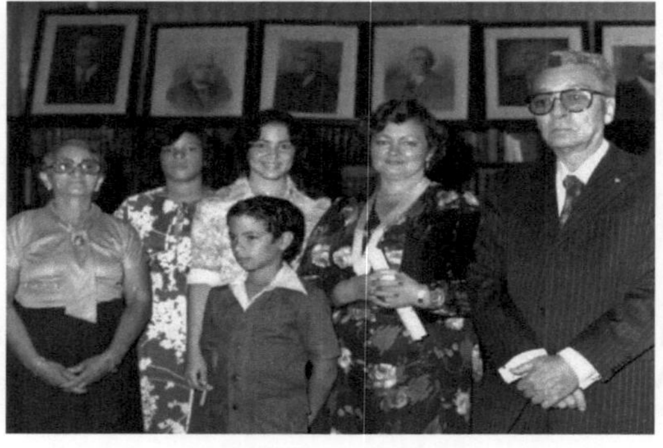

Dr. Haydée Viloria de Castejón receives from Dr. Luis Borges Duarte, President of the Academy of Medicine of Zulia, the Diploma of the Adolfo D'Empaire Prize awarded to Dr. Orlando Castejón for his work on human cerebral oedema. Present are Elba Sandoval de Castejón, Haydée Viloria de Castejón and our children Orlhay Beatriz, Heidi Cristina and Clemente Luis Castejón (1976). Dr. Castejón was in Germany participating in the Congress of the International Federation of Electron Microscopy Societies, in which he was an active researcher and a member of the International Federation of Electron Microscopy Societies. As Representative of the Society Latin American Society of Electron

Microscopy, Member Society of the International Federation.

Participation in the Organisation of the Ibero-American Society of Cell Biology. Santiago de Chile (1974)

Following the creation of the Latin American Electron Microscopy Society, a group of prominent Latin American scientists, including Drs. Ricardo Martínez Rodríguez (Spain), Jaime Pereda Tapiol and Juan de Vial (Chile), Eduardo de Robertis, Guillermo Jaim Etcheberry, Pecci Saavedra, Amanda Pellegrini de Iraldi (Argentina), Juan Kouri (Cuba), Carlos Junkeira and Wanderlay Sousa (Brazil) and José Antonio Serrano, Haydée Viloria de Castejón and Orlando Castejón (Venezuela) founded the Ibero-American Society of Cell Biology in Santiago de Chile during the II Latin American Congress of Electron Microscopy in Santiago de Chile in 1974.

The holding of the 1st Ibero-American Congress of Histochemistry and Cytochemistry, the 3rd Ibero-American Congress of Cell Biology and the 6th Latin-American Congress of Electron Microscopy (Maracaibo, Venezuela) (1984).

These congresses were held with the active participation of Dr. Haydée Viloria de Castejón and Dr. María Elena Viloria Ocando, who worked in Maracaibo at the Biological Research Unit while Dr. Orlando Castejón was Minister of Environment and Renewable Natural Resources in Caracas (1984). Dr. Viloria de Castejón and Dr. María Elena Viloria created an Organising Committee that allowed them to lead the organisation of three congresses simultaneously, which meant intensive days of organisational work. These congresses were the I Iberoamerican Congress of Histochemistry and Cytochemistry, the III Iberoamerican Congress of Cell Biology and the VI Latin American Congress of Electron Microscopy.Dr. Haydée Viloria de Castejón organised and participated as President of the 1st Iberoamerican Congress of Histochemistry and Cytochemistry held in Maracaibo, Venezuela (1984).

Photo of the Presidium of the I Iberoamerican Congress of Histochemistry and Cytochemistry. Maracaibo 1984.

Iberoamericano de Histoquimica y Citoquimica
MARACAIBO, VENEZUELA DEL 2 AL 8 DICIEMBRE 1984
III CONGRESO IBEROAMERICANO DE BIOLOGIA CELULAR
VI CONGRESO LATINOAMERICANO DE MICROSCOPIA ELECTRONICA
ORLANDO J CASTEJON HAYDEE V CASTEJON PRESIDENTES
Maracaibo, Venezuela 2-8 Diciembre 1984

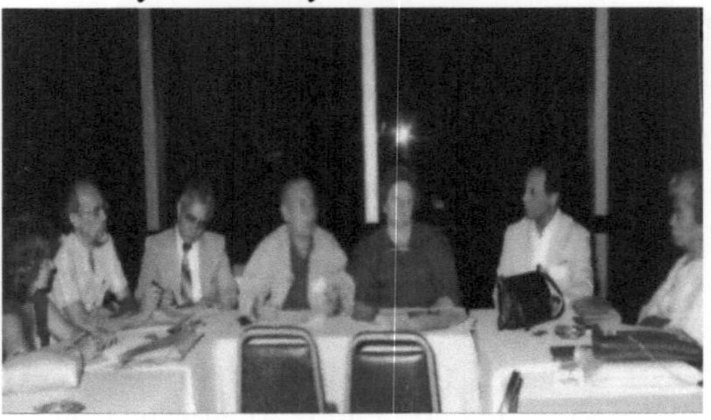

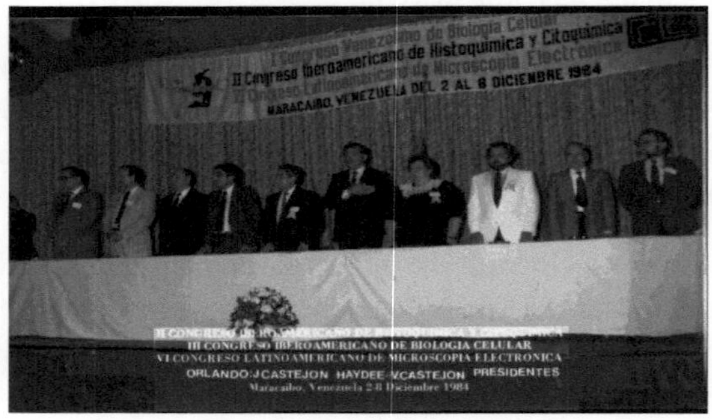

Presidium of the International Congresses integrated from left to right by Dr. Boris Drujan, Director IVIC, Ricardo Martínez Rodríguez (Spain), President of the III Iberoamerican Congress, José Antonio Serrano, Haydée Viloria de Castejón (President of the Congresses), Ángel Zambrano, Governor of Zulia State, Orlando Castejón, José Chiquinquirá Ferrer, Rector of LUZ, Humberto Fernández Morán (USA), Ramón Piezzi (Universidad del Cuyo, Argentina) and Raimundo Villegas (Director IDEA). Dr. Castejón, President of the VI Latin American Congress of Electron Microscopy, presented the keynote speech (Maracaibo, Venezuela, 1984).

Participation of Dr. Haydée Viloria de Castejón in the Ibero-American Congress of Cell Biology organised by Dr. Ricardo Martínez Rodríguez in Madrid (1987).

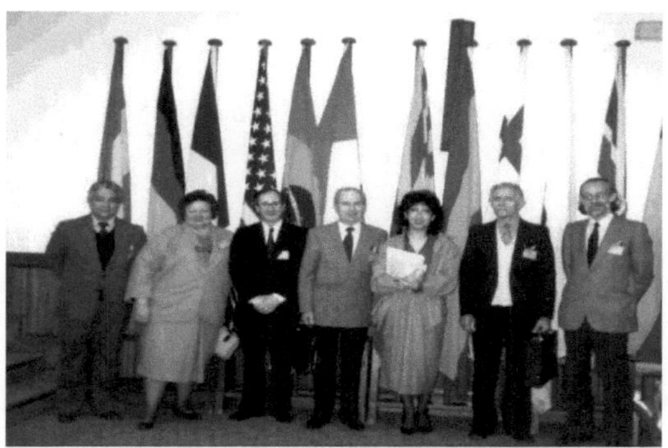

Members of the Presidium of the Ibero-American Congress of Cell Biology. Distinguished from left to right are Drs. Orlando and Haydée Castejón, José Russo, Ricardo Martínez Rodríguez, and Members of the Organising Committee in Madrid (1987).

CHAPTER VIII
ACADEMIC TRAVEL REPORTS ON THE OCCASION OF PARTICIPATION IN INTERNATIONAL CONGRESSES TRAVEL TO PARIS IN TRANSIT TO TOKYO (JAPAN)

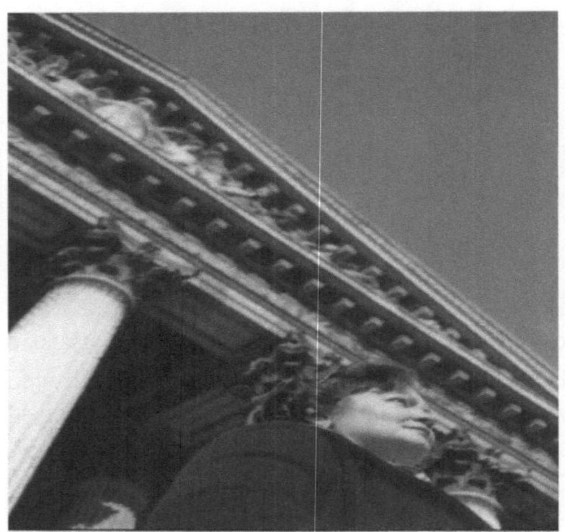

Travel to Tokyo

Dr. Viloria de Castejón was very happy contemplating the temples we visited and very excited when she presented her findings. The unceasing effort of her work over the years was being presented for the first time to the guests present who were part of her bibliographic references. She went to This generates a special tension when presenting a paper in front of cited authors who are part of the world literature.Outside congress hours we visited the shopping centres. Haydee took a special delight in pearls. She brought them to Maracaibo in a luxurious necklace as a souvenir and wore them frequently in the laboratory. She was curious about the typical Japanese dresses and bought a small kimono for our daughter Julia Aurora. In short, it was an extraordinary journey that imbued us spiritually and scientifically.

Dr. Castejón in front of a Japanese temple in Kyoto (1972) on the occasion of her participation in the IV International Congress of Histochemistry, held in Kyoto, Japan, 20-26 August 1972, where she presented the GABOUL Method for the intraneuronal detection of proteoglycans by transmission electron microscopy.

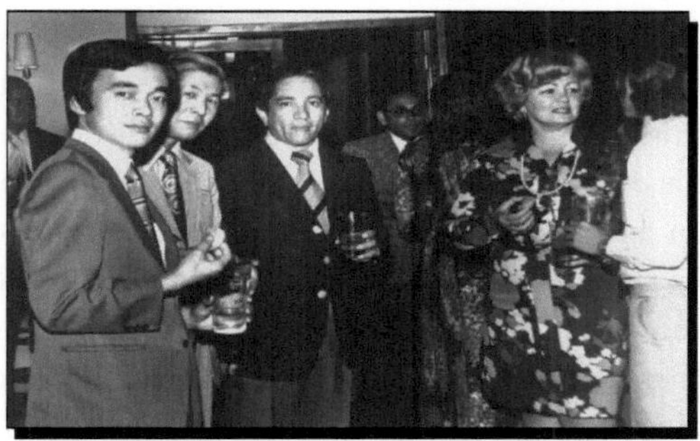

Meeting with President Susumi Ito of the Jeol Company in Japan, from whom the JEOL100B electron microscope was purchased. This The meeting was highly congenial. The President in his office displayed the Venezuelan and Japanese flags on his desk. At the Jeol we had the opportunity to see the ultra-high voltage electron microscope of one million electron volts and a size equivalent to a three-storey building.

Trip to New Orleans USA (1973).

At this 1973 American Society for Microscopy Meeting we present a paper on an electron dense stain, Ruthenium Red, for the electron microscopic demonstration of intraneuronal polysaccharides, methodology designed by Dr. Haydee Viloria de Castejón and in collaboration with Dr. María Elena Viloria.

(Haydee V. Castejón, María E. Viloria and Indalecio Rivero, Orlando Castejón: Contribution of Ruthenium Chloride to the ultracytochemical study of cerebellar cortex. Proc. XXXI Annual. Electron Microscopy Society of America. J. Arcceneau (Ed) New Orleans, USA. 1973, pp. 30-31.Haydee Viloria de Castejón's creative activity was manifested in trying to demonstrate by electron-histochemical methods the presence of proteoglycans inside nerve cells, one of her contributions.his contribution is set out in the book published by Dr. Haydee Viloria de Castejón and Dr. María Viloria. His contribution is reflected in the book published by Dr. Haydee Viloria de Castejón and Dr. María Viloria in 1977-1979 entitled Manual de Técnicas Histoquímicas (Manual of Histochemical Techniques). Her work appears in international books and monographs, such as the book on Complex Carbohydrates in Nervous Tissue published by Richard Margolis in 1979 (USA), where it is stated that Dr. Castejón made the discovery of intracytoplasmic proteoglycans in nerve cells.(See reference: The Complex carbohydrates in Nervous Tissue. Margolis R (Ed). Springer. **Plenum Press, New York** 1979. **10.1007/978-1-4613-2925-1.** Trip to Sao Paulo Brazil (1974).

We travelled to Sao Paulo in the company of my wife, Dr Haydee Viloria de Castejón, at the invitation of the Brazilian Society of Electron Microscopy to participate with several papers together with our research fellows in the incipient Biological Research Unit, Dr María Elena Viloria and Dr Consuelo Valero at the II Latin American Congress of Electron Microscopy in Ribeirao Preto in the first week of December 1974.

See the following references

1. Castejón, Orlando J. and Castejón, Haydée V. Cytochemistry and Ultrastructure of mouse and human cerebellar Golgi cells. II Latin American Congress of Electron Microscopy. Ribeirao Preto, Sao Paulo, Brazil. December 1-5th, 1974.

2. Castejón, Haydée; Castejón, Orlando J.; Viloria, Maria E. and Valero Consuelo. Ultracytochemical study of mouse cerebellar proteoglycans. Effect of methylation and enzymatic digestions. II Latin American Congress of Electron Microscopy. Ribeirao Preto. Sao Paulo. Brasil. Dicember 1-5th, 1974.

3 Viloria, Maria E.; Castejón, Haydée V.; Castejón, Orlando J. and Valero,

Consuelo. Different types of subsurface cisterns in mice and human central nervous system. II Latin American Congress of Electron Microscopy. Ribeirao Preto. Sao Paulo. Brasil. Dicember 1-5th, 1974.
4. Valero, Consuelo; Castejón, Orlando J.; Castejón, Haydée V., Viloria, Maria E.: Electron microscopic study of perifocal edema associated to human brain tumors. II Latin American Congress of Electron Microscopy. Riberao Preto. Sao Paulo. Brasil. Dicember 1-5th, 1974.

Trip to Bucharest, Romania, (1976)

In 1976 Dr. Haydée Viloria de Castejón travelled to Bucharest (Romania) accompanied by our daughters Orlhay and Beatriz and Heidi Cristina. Romania was a poor country in Europe belonging to the so-called Soviet orbit. There, they met many European participants at the 5th International Congress of Histochemistry and Cytochemistry. At this congress, Dr. Castejón presented a new method to visualise intraneuronal proteoglycans under the electron microscope. The method is called GABOUL, an abbreviation corresponding to the initials of glutaraldehyde, osmium, uranyl and lead, the names of the reagents and electronic stains used. On her return Dr. Castejón reported on the kind attention of the Romanian researchers and that of Dr. Ricardo Martínez Rodríguez, a distinguished researcher in Histochemistry at the Cajal Institute in Madrid. Since then we have maintained a close friendship that led them to organise the Ibero-American Congress of Cell Biology in Madrid in 1987. The GABOUL method was published in Acta Histochemica (Germany), and in the Proceedings of the American Microscopical Society, and in Histochemistry and Cytochemistry.

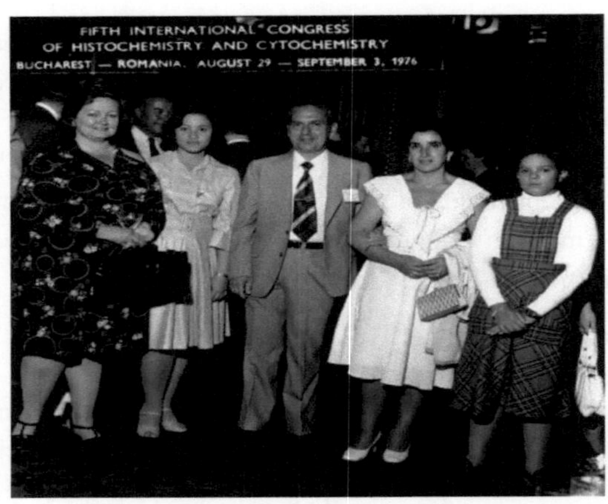

Dr Haydée Viloria de Castejon accompanied by our daughters Orlhay and Heidi and Dr Martínez Rodríguez and his wife (1976) participants in the Fifth International Congress of Histochemistry and Cytochemistry in Romania (Budapest). 1976.

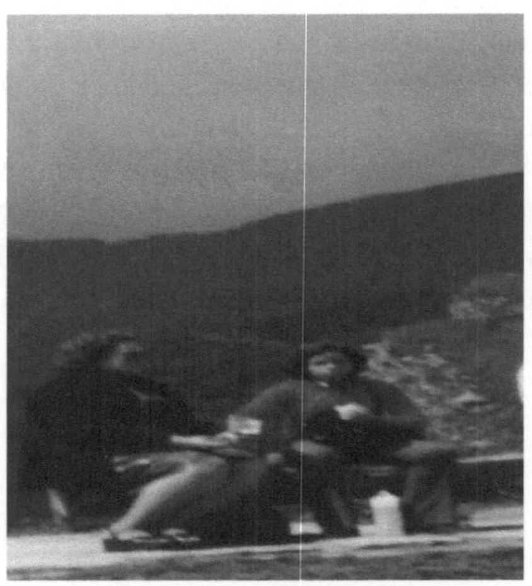

Dr. Castejón accompanied by her daughter Heidi Cristina Heidi Cristina, resting after a long walk. Romania (1976). Haydée had great sympathy for the poor countries of the Soviet orbit. On her return she commented on the enormous difficulties faced by Romanian researchers. Comments that in the impoverished Venezuela of today in which we write this trip have a profound identity.

Dr Haydee Viloria de Castejon in front of the Colosseum in Rome (1981) on a transitory journey to Zurich.

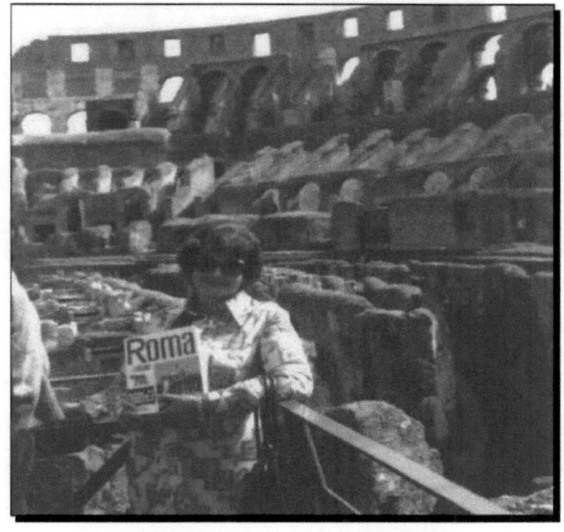

Journey to Zurich (1982)

In 1982 we travelled with my wife Haydée and my daughter Julia Aurora to Zurich to attend the First World Congress of the International Brain Organisation to be held in Zurich (Switzerland) and to present a new finding, the formation of transendothelial channels formed by endothelial cells of cerebral capillaries in severe traumatic human cerebral oedema. This work was subsequently published in Pathology Research and Practice in Germany.We took advantage of our stay to visit Professor Hans Moore at the Federal Institute of Technology in Zurich. Professor Moore had been in Maracaibo in 1972 to attend the 1st Latin American Congress of Electron Microscopy and we had established a great friendship especially after his post-congress stay at Adicora. Moore invited us to his house on the outskirts of Zurich surrounded by colourful cattle farms. Professor Moore developed the cryofracture technique for transmission electron microscopy that allowed the trilamellar structure of the membrane to be visualised and a macromolecular array to be visualised. This technique led to the interpretation of the mosaic model of the membrane as an advance on Robertson's membrane unit. Moore is an amateur photographer and proudly showed me the pictures he had taken at Adicora.He told me that when he retired he would take up photography. After lunch we took the attached photograph.

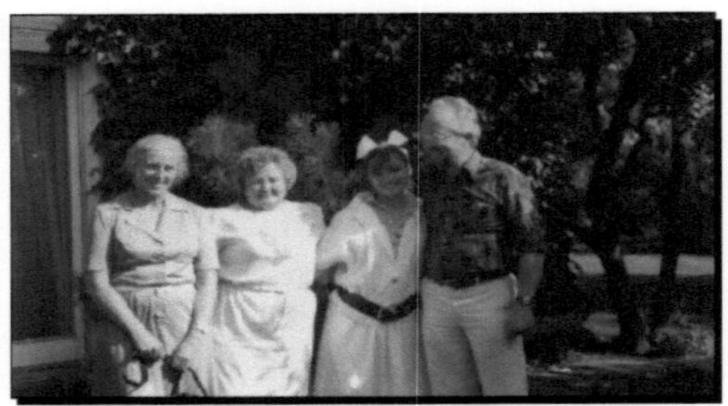

Dr. Hans Moore and his wife with Haydee and Julia Aurora at their home outside Zurich, 1982.

First Congress of the Ibero-American Federation of Histochemistry and Cytochemistry in Madrid (1987). This congress was organised by the Ibero-American Federation of Cell Biology chaired by Dr. Ricardo Martínez Rodríguez, President and Dr. Haydée Viloria de Castejón, Vice-President.

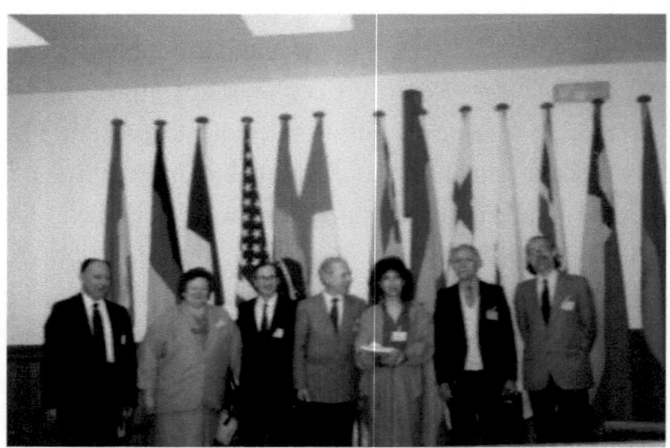

Members of the Presidium of the Ibero-American Congress of Cell Biology. Distinguished from left to right are Drs. Orlando and Haydée Castejón, José Russo, Ricardo Martínez Rodríguez, and Members of the Organising Committee in Madrid.

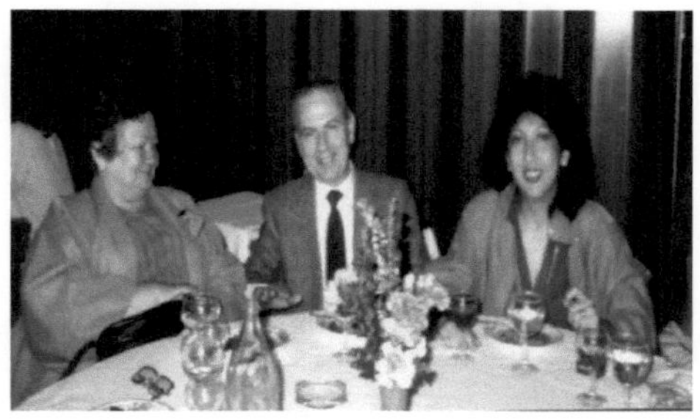

Dr Viloria de Castejón accompanied by Dr Ricardo Martínez Rodríguez during the Congress Dinner.

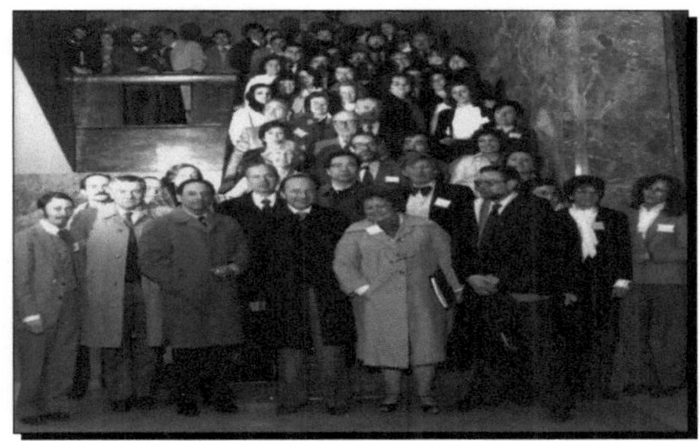

Group of participants in the Ibero-American Congress of Histochemistry and Cytochemistry (1987).

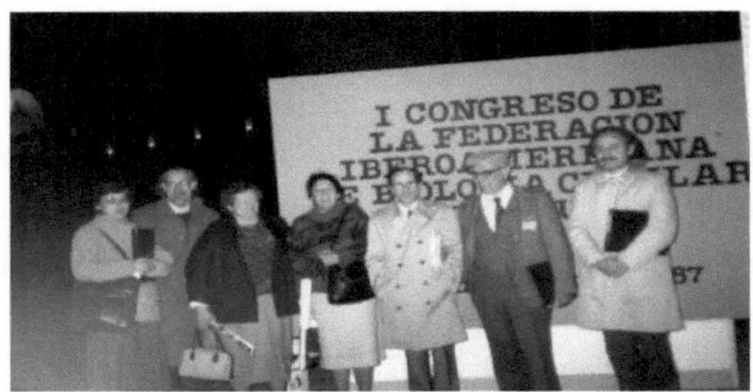

Participants in el Iberoamerican of Histochemistry and Cytochemistry. Madrid (1987)

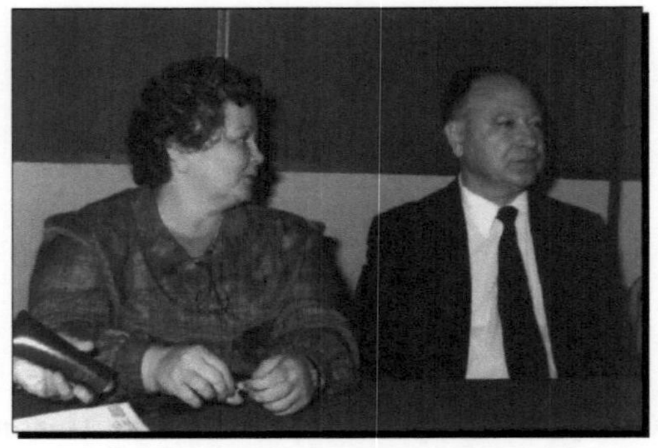

Dr Haydée Viloria de Castejon chairing a Working Table with Dr Humberto Fernández Moran (1987).

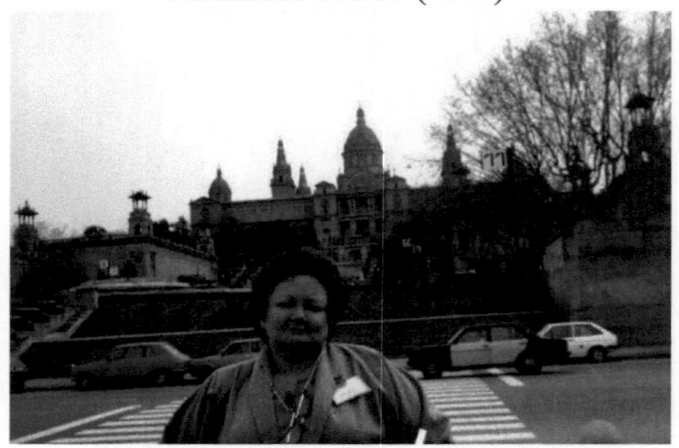

Dr Viloria de Castejón during her visit to the Prado Museum. Trip to Constance, Germany (1985)

Constance is a German city named after Emperor Constantine I the Great. Located on the southern shore of Lake Constance and bordering Switzerland, fed by the Rhine River, its pleasant climate makes it a prestigious tourist destination. Constance is historically important because Frederick I, also known as Red Beard, signed a peace with the Lombards in the early 15th century, historically known as the Peace of Constance. One of the most important tourist sites is the city centre where you can see two medieval towers, and two squares, Markstätte and Münsterplatz. A visit to the Church of Our Lady with different Romanesque, Gothic and Baroque styles testifying to the different periods of Roman and French domination of the city is mandatory.

The island of Mainau (or flower island) and Reichenau, whose monastery is a UNESCO World Heritage Site.Together with Dr. Haydee Viloria de Castejón, we were excited to present a paper on cryofracture of the cerebellar cortex using transmission microscopy and platinum carbon monoatomic metallic replicas. This technique allowed us to visualise the macromolecular configuration of neuronal membranes and to interpret them according to the studies carried out by our friend Professor Hans Moor at the Federal Institute of Technology in Zurich. Hans Moor had been in Maracaibo attending the I Latin American Congress of Electron Microscopy in 1972 which we had organised in Maracaibo. By studying his publications we learned to interpret the two characteristic phases offered by the technique, the protoplasmic phase and the extracellular phase. I remember the unforgettable meetings of Hans Moor and Fernández Moran in our flat exchanging impressions of their electron microscopy studies in impeccable German, sometimes accompanied by Peter Giebresch, Director of the Robert Koch Institute in Germany. I remember it as one of the most interesting times in my academic career to be able to discuss the scientific and technological system with some of the world's leading inspirational minds. Hans Moor had enjoyed the Congress immensely and decided to stay and join us to meet Adicora. He was a specialist in photography and was enraptured by the view of the Médanos and the blue Caribbean Sea. My Lady Haydée enjoyed the congress and the city extraordinarily. She fully identified with the scenery, the traditional dresses of the population, music and flowers. Watching her, I thought I was meeting her genes and her behaviours, which were expressed in her intelligence, her strictness, her authoritarian character and her beautiful green eyes.The presented work was subsequently published describing different aspects of cerebellar cells in specialised journals such as the European Journal of Cell Biology, Neuroscience Letters (USA) and Electron microscopy in Japan. One of the most important souvenirs was to bring back replicas of beer mugs used in the 18th century, which are displayed as part of the decoration of our bar in the flat.

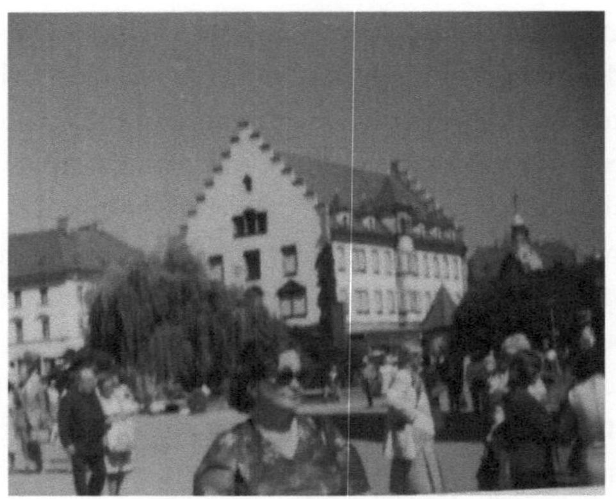

Dr. Haydée Viloria de Castejón in the Central Park of Constanza (1985)

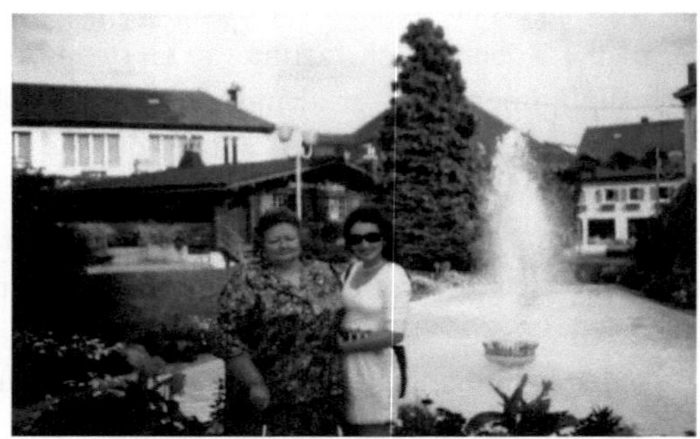

Dr Haydée Viloria de Castejón accompanied by our daughter Julia Aurora Castejón Viloria in front of the Guest House in Constanza.

Family trip to Geneva (Switzerland) to visit her husband Dr. Orlando Castejón. In Geneva (1994) accompanying her husband as Venezuela's Representative to the United Nations. During the month of August 1994 Dr. Castejón and my mother Elba Sandoval Pérez visited us in Geneva where Dr. Castejón was the Venezuelan Representative to the United Nations (UN).

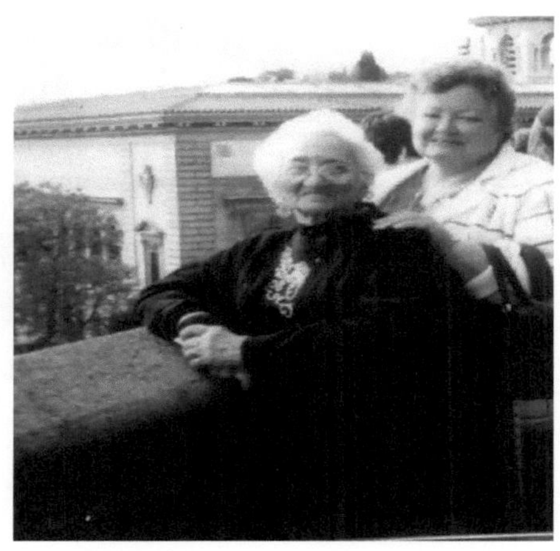

Doña Elba and Haydée in Geneva during a short holiday stay and whose farewell on their return to Venezuela gave me deep moments of inconsolable meditation (1994).

Presence of Dr. Castejón at the launching of the book Scanning Microscopy of Cerebellar Cortex by the University Authorities of the University of Zulia. Maracaibo. Venezuela

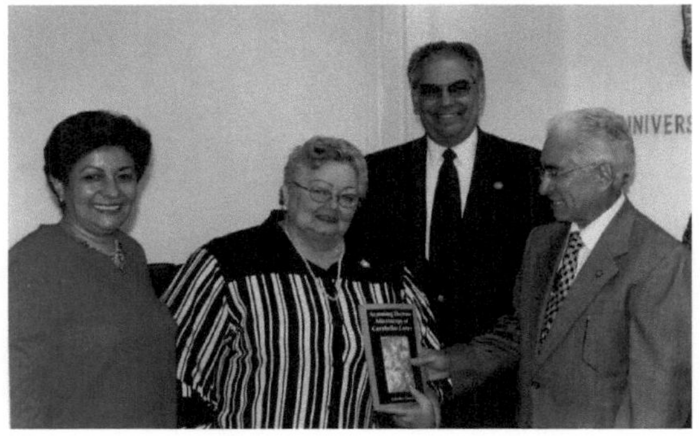

Baptism of the book Scanning Microscopy of Cerebellar Cortex by Dr. Orlando Castejón, but with Drs. Domingo Bracho and Dr. Teresita Álvarez de Fernández, Rector and Academic Vice-Rector of the University of Zulia (2002), accompanied by Dr. Alan Castellanos, Dr. Pablo Ortega and Nelly Montiel (2002). Dr. Alan Castellanos, Dr. Pablo Ortega and Nelly Montiel (2002).

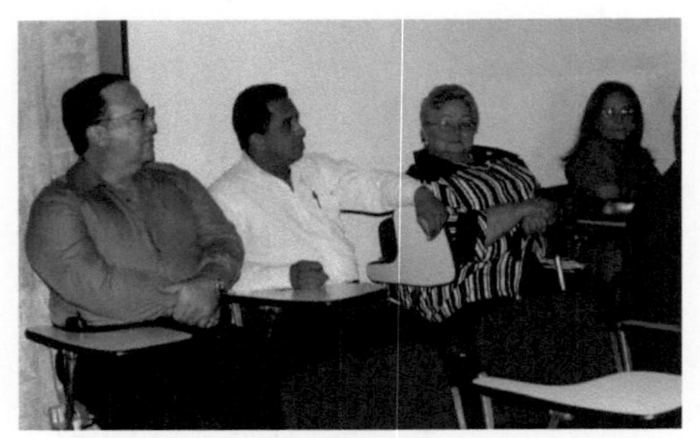

CHAPTER IX

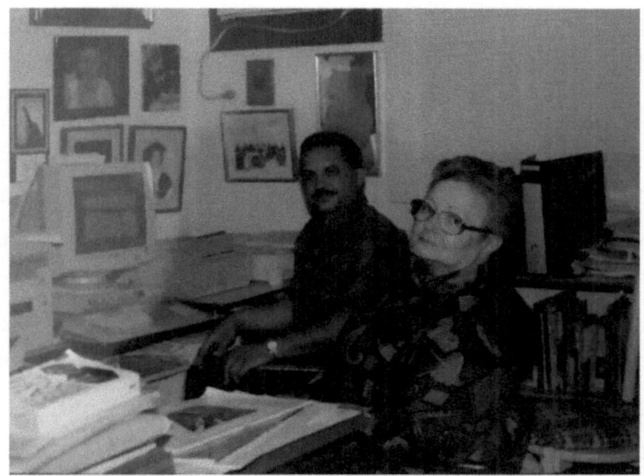

Profile of Dr. Haydée Viloria de Castejón according to De. Pablo Ortega, The Researcher in Child Malnutrition and its Social Content. "An extraordinary experience".

By Dr. Pablo Ortega, Autonomous Researcher, former Director of the Institute of Biological Research and Coordinator of the Malnutrition Programme of social impact, constituting a clear testimony of life, of the important role played by researchers in the basic sciences, when they are projected to the solution of the fundamental problems of our society.Dr. Haydée Viloria de Castejón, my Academic Tutor, not only spent time and effort in research on deficiency problems during childhood, but also focused on the search for plausible solutions. to these problems, through the multidisciplinary training of human resources, both for research and for the medical, nutritional, psychological and social care of the affected child population. These facts will be referenced throughout this chapter with his multiple participations in scientific congresses and publications in peer-reviewed scientific journals. In addition, he actively participated in the creation of institutional structures, both for research and for multidisciplinary assistance for these problems.Based on the findings of an important part of his research work in the basic sciences, and extrapolating his reflections and conclusions on the possible alterations that could occur during the different stages of growth and development of human beings, he became increasingly interested in child malnutrition and its devastating effects on the future of this population in the development of our developing society.His praiseworthy work in the scientific and welfare approach to child malnutrition began in the mid 80's, when he started an extension programme on Child Malnutrition and Mental Retardation, attached to the Institute of Biological Research of the Faculty of Medicine of our Illustrious University of Zulia, He managed to bring together a select team of professors and undergraduate and postgraduate students from the Schools of Medicine, Nutrition and Bioanalysis, whose names and outstanding participation are reflected as authors and co-authors of multiple participations in National and International Scientific Events, published in the proceedings of these events and in high impact peer-reviewed scientific journals.The impact of her teaching, research and extension activities is reflected in a short time, when she actively participates in the creation and foundation of the first Nutritional Education and Recovery Service (SERN) in the Zulia region, located in the Chiquinquira Hospital in Maracaibo, being appointed as Research Coordinator and member of the steering committee of the Service since its creation in 1987.To better understand Dr. Haydee's futuristic vision of the problem of child malnutrition and its devastating effects on growth and development during the first stages of life, we must bear in mind that in the 1970s and 1980s, Venezuela was in the midst of a socio-economic oil bonanza and the clinical pictures of child malnutrition that were presented were few and the compromise of the child's growth and development was mild to moderate. References to severe cases at that time were isolated and came from very marginal or rural areas, and from bibliographical references from very poor countries on the African continent.In 1995, with the consolidation of different lines of research and their respective programmes of action, on deficiencies of essential amino acids, vitamin A, trace elements such as zinc and iron, and based on the premise that "malnourished children present organic and functional alterations, which merit special handling by trained personnel, and that it was also necessary to continue research in order to achieve treatment alternatives that would allow their serious health problems to be dealt with effectively and in a timely manner"; requested the Technical Council of the Institute of Biological Research to create the Laboratory for Research on Childhood Malnutrition and Mental Retardation, to which a physical space was assigned, with the necessary laboratory equipment, administrative, technical and academic staff. This consolidates the local, national and international projection of the scientific and welfare activities developed so far. With this platform for action, it promotes strategic partnerships with the School of Psychology of the Rafael Urdaneta University and the Technological Park of the University of Zulia, thus multiplying the efforts in the scientific and welfare approach to the problem.There are multiple causes that combine to create the favourable conditions that give rise to child malnutrition, the main ones being: the lack or inadequate intake of nutrients in a being in full growth and development, parental ignorance, illiteracy, unemployment, poverty, overcrowding, lack of basic services. In this sense, Dr. Haydée, promoted and participated in the planning and execution of research work and activities of scientific relevance, which stood out in the field of nutritional, anthropometric and dietetic evaluation, clinical evaluation, biochemical evaluation: highlighting the studies in Glucosaminoglycans, Proteins, Amino acids, Vitamin zinc, serum Iron and Anaemias (62-69), psychological evaluation of social action and nutritional intervention.Regarding the scientific and health care approach to the problem of malnutrition in the early stages of life, not only the infant and school population was addressed in various educational centres and soup kitchens in the region (85-87), but also adolescents with nutritional deficiencies during pregnancy, in the high-risk obstetric consultation of the Gynaecology and Obstetrics Services of the Chiquinquirá Hospital and the "Dr. Armando Castillo Plaza" Maternity Hospital (88-95). Finally, as research coordinator and member of the SERN Steering Committee, she kept a watchful eye on the monitoring and updating of the various criteria and protocols for nutritional intervention in hospitalised children. The dissemination of the intervention programmes was a constant motivational factor until the last days of her life, maintaining as a central axis the Welfare Services and their expansion to other localities in the Zuliana region, in different modalities, advocating the semi-inpatient modality for marginal urban and rural areas.

"The monitoring of nutritional programmes requires political will for the effective distribution of financial, material, human and administrative resources to achieve their optimal benefit for the needy population, the future labour and intellectual future of Venezuela".
Dr. Haydée V. Castejón

CHAPTER X

Opinion of her relatives A Wise Teacher Orlhay Castejón Viloria Daughter of Haydée Viloria de Castejón and Orlando Castejón Degree in Business Administration. Specialist in Finance.

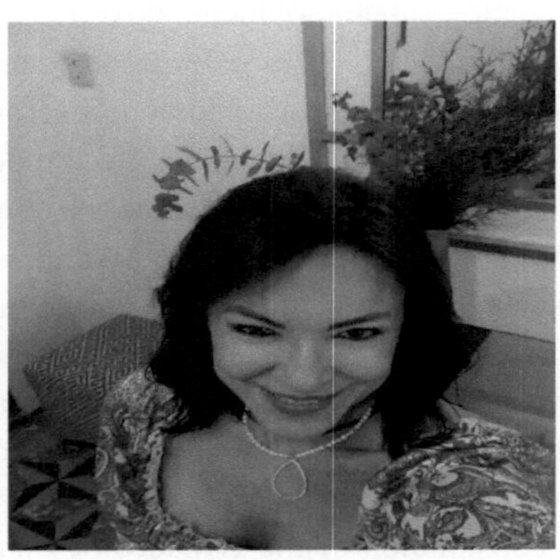

I lived and enjoyed a series of teachings from a wise teacher, a person who was rigid and accurate in her advice, from whom I inherited her capacity for leadership, organisation and planning at work, her taste for the area and her investments. She told me daughter, with effort, savings and perseverance, achievements are obtained, in silence, step by step. My best memories, her dedication and love to her children, husband, mother and her great Viloria family.Ocando. She was a selfless and tireless worker, an untiring teacher with her students in the laboratory and passionate about scientific research. She was a brilliant mind, a prolific writer in biomedical research, recognised by her international peers with whom she dialogued on her numerous national and international trips, as has been well described in this monograph. She loved her work in the area of child malnutrition and her identification with many children from our underprivileged classes. She had a long academic career, which she left her mark in the best international journals and congresses of her speciality, together with her large group of young people who accompanied her. As a loving friend and mother, she was my ally with whom I always counted on, a strong character in our social and family behaviour and always by our side. So much to thank you for your infinite virtues, for your guidance on our journeys, my beautiful old lady, you will always be present in every act of my life, spirit, mind and heart.

Dr. Julia Aurora Castejón Viloria, daughter of Dr. Haydée Viloria de Castejón
Medical Surgeon, specialist in Ophthalmology

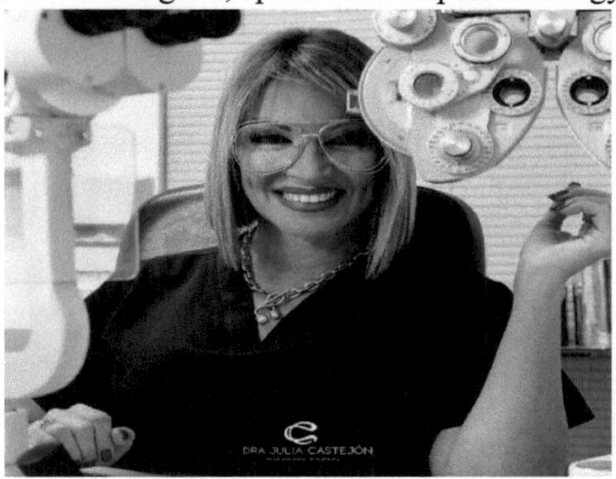

WHO WAS MY MOTHER?

Dr. Julia Aurora Castejón Viloria, another daughter of Dr. Haydée Viloria de Castejón Physician-Surgeon, specialist in Ophthalmology Without fear of being mistaken, one of the most virtuous women in the eyes of God that I have ever known. And not because she was my mother, but because her courage, effort, discipline, character, temperance, obedience, love and fear of God were sublime e unquestionable. Exceptional woman, wife and mother, unconditional, dreamer, visionary. Strict, rigorous, meticulous, studious, academically brilliant! With a drive, dynamism and energy that went beyond her physical and spiritual-physical health...The sky was the limit to reach her incredible and fruitful achievements at a level national level e international level. Dr. Haydee Viloria de Castejón; known as THE WOMAN WITH JADE EYES because of the Aqua green of her eyes. Medical Research Scientist, Head of the Histochemistry and Cytochemistry Laboratory of the Institute of Biology. Biological Researcher of the Faculty of Medicine of the Illustrious University of Zulia; leader in research programmes on child malnutrition; Founder of the Child Malnutrition Unit of the Chiquinquira Hospital, Maracaibo, Zulia State, Venezuela. A tireless mother, devoted to her children, to our school work, trades, hobbies, entrepreneurship and university studies. She encouraged us in everything we wanted to innovate and more! She facilitated, paved the way for us, her children, to be formed as human beings filled with the Holy Spirit of God and as honest, honest, capable, responsible and ethical workers! As a daughter? A loving daughter and a mother to her 9 siblings, as she was the "eldest" and my grandmother was widowed very young; she became the right hand of my maternal grandmother and together with her they managed to "raise", raise and educate the offspring. He loved his mother madly and honoured her abundantly in life, all his life!As a wife? A devoted, loyal, faithful, accomplice, friend, submissive, "enamoricienta" wife. She was the girlfriend, wife and lover of the man who captivated her heart and filled it with love and infinite admiration, she was, together with my father, co-participant and creator of an unprecedented empire and academic legacy! Mamita, 18 years ago heaven and earth opened to receive you, the purifying fire and a bed of white roses were laid out ...your ascent was heartfelt, fragrant, beautiful.I remember hearing in the distance, the chords of "Alfonsina y el Mar" sung with emotion and tears by my adorable sister Heidi Cristina as we anguishedly said goodbye to you amidst tears and restless silent choking... Earthly precocious your absence ?...Papa God is not wrong! Such a virtuous angel should be in the heavenly gardens dancing with the A gels of God! Love, sacrifice, detachment, what teachings Mamita!I honour you and thank you for the love beyond measure. We love and miss you forever and ever. Blessing!

CHAPTER XI

COMMUNICATIONS TO CONGRESSES AND PUBLICATIONS BY DR HAYDÉE VILORIA DE CASTEJÓN AND COLLABORATORS

1) Castejón, Haydée V.; Castejón, Orlando J. and Viloria, María E.: Application of GABOUL technique in the electron microscopy study of mouse and human cerebral cortex nerve cells. Histochemistry and Cytochemistry. pp. 69-70, 1970.

2) Haydée V. Castejón, Orlando J. Castejón and R. Romero Rincón...: Histochemical and ultrastructural study of the liver cell in a case of type I glycogenosis. Invest. Clín. 38: 9-49, 1971.

3) Haydée V. Castejón, Orlando J. Castejón and R. Romero Rincón...: Histochemical and ultrastructural study of the liver cell in a case of type I glycogenosis. Invest. Clín. 38: 9-49, 1971.

4) Haydée V. Castejón and Orlando J. Castejón: Application of Alcian Blue and Osmium- Dimethylothylenediamine (Os-DMEDA) in the electronhistochemical study of nerve tissue. Proceedings of Histochemistry. pp. 519-520, 1972.

5) Haydée V. Castejón and Orlando J. Castejón: Application of Alcian Blue and Os- DMEDA in the electron histochemical study of cerebellar cortex. I. Alcian Blue staining. Symposium on Fine Structure of Cerebellum. Rev. Micr. Elec. Vol. 1, No. 2: 207-226. 1972.

6) Orlando J. Castejón and Haydée V. Castejón: Application of Alcian Blue and Os- DMEDA in the electron histochemical study of cerebellar cortex. II. Os-SMEDA staining. Symposium on Fine Structure of Cerebellum. Rev. Micr. Elec. Vol. 1, No. 2: 227-238. 1972

7) Haydée V. Castejón and Orlando J. Castejón : Application of Alcian Blue and Osmium- Dimethylothylenediamine (Os-DMEDA) in the electronhistochemical study of nerve tissue. Proc Histochem. pp. 519-520, 1972.

8) Haydée V. Castejón and Orlando J. Castejón. Application of Alcian Blue and Os-DMEDA in the electron histochemical study of cerebellar cortex. I. Alcian Blue staining. Symposium on Fine Structure of Cerebellum. Rev. Micr. Elec. Vol. 1, No. 2: 207-226. 1972.

9) Orlando J. Castejón and Haydée V. Castejón: Application of Alcian Blue and Os- DMEDA in the electron histochemical study of cerebellar cortex. II. Os-SMEDA staining. Symposium on Fine Structure of Cerebellum. Rev. Micr. Elec. Vol. 1, No. 2: 227-238. 1972.

10) Orlando J. Castejón, Haydée V. Castejón, Consuelo Valero and María E. Viloria: Application of the GABOUL method to the ultracytochemical study of cerebellar capillaries. Acta Cientif. Venez. Vol. 25 (Sup. 1): 57-58, 1974.

11) Haydée V. Castejón and Orlando J. Castejón : Application of Alcian Blue and Osmium- Dimethylothylenediamine (Os-DMEDA) in the electronhistochemical study of nerve tissue. Proc Histochem. pp. 519-520, 1972.

12) Haydée V. Castejón and Orlando J. Castejón. Application of Alcian Blue and Os- DMEDA in the electron histochemical study of cerebellar cortex. I. Alcian Blue staining. Symposium on Fine Structure of Cerebellum. Rev. Micr. Elec. Vol. 1, No. 2: 207-226. 1972.

13) Orlando J. Castejón and Haydée V. Castejón: Application of Alcian Blue and Os- DMEDA in the electron histochemical study of cerebellar cortex. II. Os-SMEDA staining. Symposium on Fine Structure of Cerebellum. Rev. Micr. Elec. Vol. 1, No. 2: 227-238. 1972.

14) Haydée V. Castejón, Orlando J. Castejón and Lourdes Salazar: Ultracytochemical demonstration of hyaluronidase-sensitive acidic glycosaminoglycans in cerebellar mossy fibres. Acta Científ. Venez. 24 (Sup. 1): 47, 1973.

15) Orlando J. Castejón, Haydée V. Castejón, María E. Viloria and Indalecio Rivero: Contribution of Ruthenium Chloride to the ul-tracytochemical study of cerebellar cortex. Proceedings XXXI Annual Meeting. Electron Microscopy Society of America.J. Arcceneau (Ed) New Orleans, USA. 1973, pp. 30-31.

16) Orlando J. Castejón, Haydée V. Castejón, Consuelo Valero and María E. Viloria: Application of the GABOUL method to the ultracytochemical study of cerebellar capillaries. Acta Cientif. Venez. Vol. 25 (Sup. 1): 57-58, 1974.

17) Orlando J. Castejón and Haydée V. Castejón: The GABOUL method and its contribution to the ultracytochemical study of the cerebellar cortex. Electron Microscopy 1974. J. V. Sanders and D.J. Goodchild (Eds). Australian Academy of Science. Canberra, Australia. Vol. II, 1974, pp 328-329.

18) Orlando J. Castejón, Haydée V. Castejón, Consuelo Valero and María E. Viloria: Application of the GABOUL method to the ultracytochemical study of cerebellar capillaries. Acta Cientif. Venez. Vol. 25 (Sup. 1): 57-58, 1974.

19) Haydée V. Castejón, Orlando J. Castejón, María E. Viloria and Consuelo Valero: Ultracytochemical study of mouse cerebellar proteoglycans. Effect of methylation and enzymatic digestions. Proc. II Latin American Congress of Electron Microscopy. Bello Horizonte. Brazil: pp. 32-33, 1974.

20) Orlando J. Castejón and Haydée V. Castejón: Cytochemistry and ultrastructure of mouse and human cerebellar Golgi cells. Proc. II Congreso Latinoamericano de Microscopía Electrónica. Micros: pp. 34-35, 1974.

21) Consuelo Valero, Orlando J. Castejón, Haydée V. Castejón, María E. Viloria and José Ramón Guzmán: Electron microscopic study of perifocal edema associated to heman brain tumors. II Latin American Congress of Electron Microscopy. Bello Horizonte. Brazil. pp. 128-129,1974.

22) María E. Vilora, Haydée V. Castejón, Orlando J. Castejón and Consuelo Valero: Different types of subsurface cisterns in mice and human central nervous systems. Proc. II Latin American Congress of Electron Microscopy. Bello Horizonte. Brazil. pp. 134-135, 1974.

23) Consuelo Valero, Orlando J. Castejón, Haydée V. Castejón, María E. Viloria and José Ramón Guzmán: Electron microscopic study of perifocal edema associated to heman brain tumors. II Latin American Congress of Electron Microscopy. Bello Horizonte. Brazil. pp. 128-129,1974.

24) María E. Vilora, Haydée V. Castejón, Orlando J. Castejón and Consuelo Valero: Different types of subsurface cisterns in mice and human central nervous systems. Proc. II Congreso Latinoamericano de Microscopia Electrónica Bello Horizonte. Brazil. pp. 134-135, 1974.

25) María E. Vilora, Haydée V. Castejón, Orlando J. Castejón and Consuelo Valero: Different types of subsurface cisterns in mice and human central nervous systems. Proc. II Latin American Congress of Electron Microscopy Bello Horizonte. Brazil. pp. 134-135, 1974.

26) Castejón, Orlando J. and Castejón, Haydée V.: Application of GABOUL method to the ultracytochemical study of mouse blood-brain barrier. Proceedings Electron Microscopy Society of America. pp. 98-99, 1976.

27) Viloria, María E.; Castejón, Haydée V. and Castejón, Orlando J.: Application of Alcian Blue to the submicroscopic study of capillary cells in human brain edema. Journal of Electron Microscopy, 3: 144-145, 1976.

28) Castejón, O.J. and Castejón, H.V.: Transmission and scanning electron microscopy and ultracytochemistry of vertebrate and human cerebellar cortex. In "Glial and Neuronal Cell Biology". Ed. Sergey Federoff, pp. 249-258, Alan R. Liss, Inc. New York, 1981.
29) Castejón, O.J.; Castejón, H.V.; Alvarado, M.E.; Montiel, N.J. and Espinoza, J.R.: The cerebellar stellate neurons. A freeze-fracture and ultrastructural study. Neuroscience Letters. Suppl. 22, 271-272, 1986.
30) Castejón, O.J. and Castejón, H.V.: Electron microscopy and glycosaminoglycan histochemistry of cerebellar stellate neurons. Scanning Microscopy. 1, 681-693. 1987.
31) Castejón, O.J. and Castejón, H.V.: Scanning electron microscopy freeze etching and glycosaminoglycan cytochemical studies of the cerebellar climbing fiber system. Scanning Microscopy, 2, 2181-2193, 1988.
32) Castejón, O.J. and Castejón, H.V. Three-dimensional morphology of cerebellar protoplasmic islands and proteoglycan content in mossy fiber glomerulus: A scanning and transmission electron microscope study. Scanning Microscopy 5(2): 477-494, 1991.
33) Castejón, O.J. and Castejón, H.V. Three-dimensional morphology of cerebellar protoplasmic islands and proteoglycan content in mossy fiber glomerulus: A scanning and transmission electron microscope study. Scanning Microscopy 5(2): 477-494, 1991.
34) Castejón O.J., Castejón H.V., Apkarian R.P. High resolution (SE-1) scanning electron microscopy features of primate cerebellar cortex. Cellular and Molecular Biology, (Paris), 40 (9), 1173-1181, 1994.

35) Castejón O.J. Castejón, H.V., Apkarian R.P. Proteoglycan ultracytochemistry and conventional and high resolution scanning electron microscopy of vertebrate cerebellar parallel fiber presynaptic endings. Cellular and Molecular Biology (Paris) 40 (6), 795- 801, 1994.
36) Orlando J. Castejón, Haydée V. Castejón. Conventional and high resolution scanning electron microscopy of cerebellar Purkinje cells. Biocell, 21 (2) 149-160, 1997.
37) Castejón O.J., Castejón H.V., Apkarian R.P. High resolution (SE-1) scanning electron microscopy features of primate cerebellar cortex. Cellular and Molecular Biology, (Paris), 40 (9), 1173-1181, 1994.
38) Castejón O.J. Castejón, H.V.,Apkarian R.P. Proteoglycan ultracytochemistryand conventional and high resolution scanning electron

microscopy of vertebrate cerebrate cerebellar parallel fiber presynaptic endings. Cellular and Molecular Biology (Paris) 40 (6), 795-801, 1994.
39) Castejón O.J. Castejón, H.V., Conventional and high resolution scanning electron microscopy of cerebellar Purkinje cells. Biocell, 21 (2) 149-160, 1997
40) Castejon OJ, Castejon HV, Apkarian RP . Confocal laser scanning, conventional scanning and transmission electron microscopy of vertebrate cerebellar granule cell. Biocell, 25: 235-255. 2000
41) Castejón OJ, Castejón H.V.Oligodendroglial cell behaviour in traumatic oedematous human cerebral cortex. A light and electron microscopic study. Brain Injury, 14, 303- 317, 2000.
42) Castejón O.J. Castejón, H.V., and Sims P. Confocal, scanning and transmission electron microscopic study of cerebellar mossy fiber glomeruli. J. Submicrosc. Cytol. Pathol., 32 (2), 247-260, 2000.
43) Castejón O.J. Light microscopy and conventional and high resolution scanning electron microscopy of Golgi cells of vertebrate cerebellum. Biocell (Argentina) 24, 13-30, 2000.
44) Castejón OJ, Castejón H.V.Oligodendroglial cell behaviour in traumatic oedematous human cerebral cortex. A light and electron microscopic study. Brain Injury, 14, 303- 317, 2000.
45) Castejón O.J. Castejón, H.V., and Sims P. Confocal, scanning and transmission electron microscopic study of cerebellar mossy fiber glomeruli. J. Submicrosc. Cytol. Pathol., 32 (2), 247-260, 2000.
46) Castejón OJ, Castejón, HV. Correlative microscopy of cerebellar basket cells. Journal Submicroscopic, Cytology and Pathology, 33, 23-32, 2001.
47) Castejón O.J., Apkarian R.P., Castejón H.V. and Alvarado M.V.: Field emission scanning electron microscopy and freeze-fracture transmission electron microscopy of mouse cerebellar synaptic contacts. Journal Submicroscopic Cytology and Pathology, 33, 289-300, 2001.
48) Castejón O.J., Castejón H.V. and Castellano A.: Oligodendroglial cell damage and demyelination in infant hydrocephalus. An electron microscopy study. Journal Submicroscopic Cytology and Pathology. 33, 33-40, 2001.
49) Castejón, OJ., Castejón HV., Diaz M., and Castellano A. Consecutive light microscopy, scanning-transmission electron microscopy and transmission electron microscopy of traumatic human brain oedema and ischaemic brain damage. Histology and Histopathology. 16,1117-1134, 2001.

50) Castejón O.J. and Castejón, H.V.: Correlative microscopy of cerebellar basket cells. Journal Submicroscopic Cytology and Pathology (Italy) 33, 23-32, 2001.

51) Castejón OJ, Castejón, HV. Correlative microscopy of cerebellar basket cells. Journal Submicroscopic, Cytology and Pathology, 33, 23-32, 2001.

52) Castejón O.J., Apkarian R.P., Castejón H.V. and Alvarado M.V.: Field emission scanning electron microscopy and freeze-fracture transmission electron microscopy of mouse cerebellar synaptic contacts. Journal Submicroscopic Cytology and Pathology, 33, 289-300, 2001.

53) Castejón O.J., Castejón H.V. and Castellano A.: Oligodendroglial cell damage and demyelination in infant hydrocephalus. An electron microscopy study. Journal Submicroscopic Cytology and Pathology. 33, 33-40, 2001.

54) Castejón O.J., Castejón H.V. and Castellano A. Oligodendroglial cell damage and demyelination in infant hydrocephalus. An electron microscopy study. Journal Submicroscopic Cytology and Pathology (Italy), 33, 33-40, 2001.

55) Castejón, OJ., Castejón HV., Diaz M., and Castellano A. Consecutive light microscopy, scanning-transmission electron microscopy and transmission electron microscopy of traumatic human brain oedema and ischaemic brain damage. Histol. Histopathol (Spain). -1134, 2001.

56) Castejón, OJ., Castejón HV., Diaz M., and Castellano A. Consecutive light microscopy, scanning-transmission electron microscopy and transmission electron microscopy of traumatic human brain oedema and ischaemic brain damage. Histology and Histopathology. 16,1117-1134, 2001.

57) Castejón OJ, Castejón HV, Díaz M, Sánchez M and Zavala M. A light and electron microscoy study of edematous human cerebral cortex in two patients with post-traumatic seizures. Brain Injury, 16,331-346, 2002.

58) Castejón O.J., Díaz M., Castejón H.V. and Castellano A.: Glycogen-rich and glycogen- depleted astrocytes in the oedematous human cerebral cortex associated with brain trauma, tumours and congenital malformations: an electron microscopy study. Brain Injury, 116,109-132, 2002.

59) Castejón O.J., Dailey, M.E., Apkarian R.P. and Castejón H.V.: Correlative microscopy of cerebellar Bergmann glial cells. J. Submicroscopic. Cytology and Pathology. 34, 131-142, 2002.

60) Castejón O.J. and Castejón H.V. Correlative microscopy of cerebellar intracortical circuits. I. Mossy and climbing fibers. In: Science, Technology

and Education of Microscopy. A. Mendez Vilas (Editor). Formatex. Badajoz. Badajoz. Spain. Spain. November 2002.

61) Castejón, O.J. and Castejón, H.V. Correlative microscopy of cerebellar intrinsic circuits. In: Science, Technology and Education of Microscopy. A. Mendez Vilas (Editor). Formatez. Badajoz. Badajoz. Spain. Spain. November 2002.

62) Castejón OJ, Castejón HV, Díaz M, Sánchez M and Zavala M. A light and electron microscoy study of edematous human cerebral cortex in two patients with post-traumatic seizures. Brain Injury (England), 16, 331-346, 2002.

63) Castejón O.J., Díaz M., Castejón H.V. and Castellano A.: Glycogen-rich and glycogen- depleted astrocytes in the oedematous human cerebral cortex associated with brain trauma, tumours and congenital malformations: an electron microscopy study. Brain Injury (England), 116,109-132, 2002.

64) Castejón O.J., Dailey, M.E., Apkarian R.P. and Castejón H.V.: Correlative microscopy of cerebellar Bergmann glial cells. J. Submicroscopic. Cytol. Pathol. (Italy), 34, 131- 142, 2002.

65) Castejón OJ, Castejón HV, Díaz M, Sánchez M and Zavala M. A light and electron microscoy study of edematous human cerebral cortex in two patients with post-traumatic seizures. Brain Injury, 16,331-346, 2002.

66) 65. Castejón O.J., Díaz M., Castejón H.V. and Castellano A.: Glycogen-rich and glycogen-depleted astrocytes in the oedematous human cerebral cortex associated with brain trauma, tumours and congenital malformations: an electron microscopy study. Brain Injury, 116,109-132, 2002.

67) 66 Castejón O.J., Dailey, M.E., Apkarian R.P. and Castejón H.V.: Correlative microscopy of cerebellar Bergmann glial cells. J. Submicroscopic. Cytology and Pathology. 34, 131-142, 2002.

68) 67. Castejón O.J. and Castejón H.V. Correlative microscopy of cerebellar intracortical circuits. I. Mossy and climbing fibers. In: Science, Technology and Education of Microscopy. A. Mendez Vilas (Editor). Formatex. Badajoz. Badajoz. Spain. Spain. November 2002.

69) 68. Castejón, O.J. and Castejón, H.V. Correlative microscopy of cerebellar intrinsic circuits. In: Science, Technology and Education of Microscopy. A. Mendez Vilas (Editor). Formatez. Badajoz. Badajoz. Spain. Spain. November 2002.

Communications to congresses

70) Orlando J. Castejón and Haydée V. de Castejón. Fixation of the mouse central nervous system by vascular perfusion with glutaraldehyde. XVI Annual ASOVAC Convention. Caracas, May, 1966.
71) 2 Haydée V. Castejón and Orlando J. Castejón. Histochemistry of intraneuronal acid mucopolysaccharides. XVI Annual Convention of ASOVAC. May, 1966. Caracas.

72) 3. Castejón, Haydée V.; Castejón, Orlando J. and Viloria, María E.: Application of GABOUL technique in the electron microscopy study of mouse and human cerebral cortex nerve cells. Histochemistry and Cytochemistry. pp. 69-70, 1970.
73) 4. Castejón, Haydée V. and Orlando J. Castejón. Application of Alcian Blue and Osmium Dimethylethylenediamine (Os-DMEDA) in the electron histochemical study of nerve tissue. Invited Speaker. IV International Congress of Histochemistry. Kyoto, Japan. 20- 26 August 1972.
74) Castejón, Haydée V.; Castejón, Orlando J. and Salazar Lourdes. Ultracytochemical demonstration of hyaluronidase-sensitive acidic glycosaminoglycans in cerebellar mucosal fibres. XXIII Annual Convention of ASOVAC. Merida, 3-7 July 1973.
75) Castejón, Orlando J., Castejón, Haydée V. and Salazar, Lourdes. The GABOUL method and its contribution to the ultracytochemical study of the cerebellar cortex. International Colloquium on Histochemistry. Tours, France. Tours, France. 1-4 July 1973.
76) . Castejón, Orlando J., Castejón, Haydée V., Viloria, Maria E. and Rivero, Indalecio. Contribution of ruthenium chloride to the ultracytochemical study of cerebellar cortex.XXXIAnnual Meeting. EMSA, and VIII Annual Meeting EPASA. New Orleans. Louisiana, U.S.A. 13-17th August. 1973.
77) Morán, Euro, González, Leonte, Castejón, Haydée V. and Castejón, Orlando J. Ultrastructural analysis of diphenylhydantoin on the mouse cerebellar cortex. XXIII Annual Convention of ASOVAC. Mérida, 3-7 July 1973.
78) González, Leonte, Morán Euro, Castejón, Haydée V. and Castejón, Orlando J. Effect of diphenylhydantoin on the mouse cerebellar cortex. X International Congress of Neurology. Barcelona, Spain. September 8-15, 1973.

79) Castejón, Orlando J. and Castejón, Haydée V. The GABOUL method and its contribution to the ultracytochemical study of the cerebellar cortex.Eigth International Congress on Electron Microscopy. Canberra, Australia, August 25-31st, 1974.

80) Castejón, Haydée V. and Castejón, Orlando J. Electronocytochemical demonstration of cerebellar cortex proteoglycans using the GABOUL method. XXIV Annual Convention of ASOVAC. Maracaibo. Maracaibo. October 7-11, 1974.

81) Castejón, Orlando J., Castejón, Haydée V., Viloria, María E. and Valero, Consuelo. Ultracytochemical demonstration of a dendritic sheath in Purkinje and Golgi cells of the cerebellar cortex. XXIV Annual Convention of ASOVAC. Maracaibo. October 7-11, 1974.

82) Castejón, Orlando J., Castejón, Haydée V., Valero, Consuelo y Viloria, María E. Application of the GABOUL method to the ultracytochemical study of cerebellar capillaries. XXIV Annual Convention of ASOVAC. Maracaibo. October 7-11, 1974.

83) Castejón, Haydée V., Viloria, María E., Castejón, Orlando J. and Valero, Consuelo. Superficial cisternae in neurons and glia of the mouse CNS. XXIV Annual Convention of ASOCAC. Maracaibo 7-11 October 1974.

84) Castejón, Orlando J. and Castejón, Haydée V. Modelo de enseñanza de la metodología de la investigación biomédica. V Pan-American Conference on Medical Education. Caraballeda. Venezuela. Caraballeda. Venezuela. 4 - 7 November 1974.

85) 1Castejón, Orlando J. and Castejón, Haydée V. Cytochemistry and Ultrastructure of mouse and human cerebellar Golgi cells. II Latin American Congress of Electron Microscopy. Ribeirao Preto, Sao Paulo, Brazil. December 1-5th, 1974.

6.Castejón, Haydée; Castejón, Orlando J.; Viloria, Maria E. and Valero Consuelo. Ultracyto chemical study of mouse cerebellar proteoglycans. Effect of methylation and enzymatic digestions. II Latin American Congress of Electron Microscopy. Ribeirao Preto. Sao Paulo. Brazil. December 1-5th, 1974.

86) Viloria, Maria E.; Castejón, Haydée V.; Castejón, Orlando J. and Valero, Consuelo. Different types of subsurface cisterns in mice and human central nervous system. II Latin American Congress of Electron Microscopy. Ribeirao Preto. Sao Paulo. Brasil. December 1-5th, 1974.

87) Valero, Consuelo; Castejón, Orlando J.; Castejón, Haydée V., Viloria, Maria E.: Electron microscopic study of perifocal edema associated to human brain tumors. II Latin American Congress of Electron Microscopy. Riberao Preto. Sao Paulo. Brasil. December 1-5th, 1974.

88) Castejón, Haydée V.; Castejón, Orlando J. and Viloria, Maria E. Application of alcian blue to the submicroscopic study of neurons in the human and mouse cerebral cortex. XXV Annual Convention of ASOVAC. Caracas, 26-31 October 1975.

89) . Castejón, Haydée V.; Castejón, Orlando J. and Viloria, Maria E. Application of Gaboul technique in the electron microscopy study of mouse and human cerebral cortex nerve cells. The Fifth International Congress of Histochemistry and Cytochemistry. Bucharest. August 29th to September 3th, 1976.

90) Castejón, Haydée V., Viloria, María E. and Castejón Orlando J.: Presence of sulphated polyanions in nerve cells of Arius spixii fish. Preliminary Communication. XXVI Annual Convention of ASOVAC. Puerto La Cruz, 7 to 13 November 1976.

91) Viloria, María E.; Castejón, Haydée V. and Castejón, Orlando J. Application of Alcian Blue to the submicroscopic study of capillary endothelial cell in human brain edema. III Latin American Congress of Electron Microscopy. Santiago (Chile) 22-26 November 1976.

92) Castejón, Orlando J.; Castejón, Haydée V. and Martínez, Esther. Design of a curricular model for a postgraduate course of Magister and Doctorate in Cellular and Molecular Biology. IV Latin American Congress of Electron Microscopy and I Iberoamerican Congress of Cell Biology. Mendoza, Argentina, 12-18 October 1978.

93) Castejón, Orlando J. and Castejón, Haydée V. Transmission electron microscopy, scanning microscopy and histochemistry of Golgi cells of the human cerebellum.

XXIX ASOVAC National Convention, Barquisimeto, Lara State. 25-30 November 1978.

94) Castejón, Orlando J.; Castejón, Haydée V. and Martínez, Esther. Design and implementation of a Postgraduate Course in Cellular and Molecular Biology. XXIX National Convention of ASOVAC. Barquisimeto, Lara State, 25-30 November 1979.

95) Castejón, Orlando J. and Castejón, Haydée V.: Transmission and

scanning electron microscopy and ultracytochemistry of vertebrate and human cerebellar cortex. XIth International Congress Anatomy. Quebec. Canada. August, 17-23rd, 1980.

96) Castejón, O.J.; Castejón, H.V. and Martínez, A.E.: Design and implementation of a postgraduate course in Cellular and Molecular Biology. VIII Meeting of Medical Education Offices. Ciudad Guyana, Venezuela. February 22-24, 1980.

97) Castejón, O.J.; Castejón, H.V.; Alvarado, M.E.; Montiel, N.; Espinoza, J.: The cerebellar stellate neurons. A freeze-fracture and ultracytochemical study by means of TEM and SEM. 9th European Meeting of the European Neuroscience Association. Ox- ford, London. September 8-12, 1985.

98) Castejón, O.J.; Castejón, H.V.; Alvarado, M.V.; Montiel, N.J. and Espinoza, J.R.: The cerebellar stellate neurons. A freeze-fracture and ultracytochemical study by means of TEM and SEM. Invited Speaker. Symposium on Scanning Electron Microscopy. New Orleans, U.S.A. May 1-4, 1986.

99) Orlando J. Castejón, Haydee V. Castejón...: Application of transmission and scanning electron microscopy to the study of the Purkinje cell of the vertebrate cerebellum. V Jornadas Científicas de la Facultad de Medicina, 23-27 September 1991. Maracaibo, Zulia State. XLI Annual Convention of ASOVAC, 24-29 November 1991.

100) Orlando J. Castejón, Haydee V. Castejón...: Further observations on scanning and transmission electron microscopy of vertebrate cerebellar Purkinje cells. Invited Speaker. Symposium on Scanning Electron Microscopy 1991. Bethesda, Maryland.
U.S.A. May 1-5th. 1991

101) Castejón, O.J.; Apkarian, R. P.; Castejón, H.V.; Sánchez, M.E.; Hernández, S.; Palmar, M.; Valero, C.; Castellano, A.; Caspersen, R.; Montiel, N.; Espinoza, R.: Examination of nerve cell surface with conventional and high-resolution SEM. A corre- lative study of gold-palladium and chromium coating samples. Scanning Meeting, Orlando, Florida, U.S.A. April, 10-14, 1993.

102) Castejón, O.J., Castejón, H.V., Díaz, M., Valero, C.: Human traumatic brain edema and cortical synaptic degeneration. 24th Annual Meeting of Society for Neuroscience. Miami, USA, November, 13-18, 1994.

103) Zavala, M., Montiel, N., Ortega, P., Borregales, L., Molano, N.,

Méndez, G.N., Urrieta, J.R., Villalobos, P.N., Castejón, O.J., Castejón, H.V.: Amino Acid Values plasmatic levels in autistic children. VII Jornadas Científicas de la Facultad Experimental de Ciencias, LUZ. July 1996.
104) Orlando J. Castejón and Haydée V. Casejón: The tintorial potentiality of two basic stains in the electron histochemical study of polyanionic compounds in nerve tissue. I. Synaptic region. Acta Histochemica (JENA). 43: 153-163, 1972.
105) Orlando J. Castejón and Haydée V. Castejón, et al: Light microscope cytochemistry and ultrastructural study of mouse cerebellar Golgi cells. Journal of Electron Microscopy. Vol. I No.1: 162-163, 1972.
106) Haydée V. Castejón and Orlando J. Castejón: Application of Alcian Blue and Osmium-Dimethylothylenediamine (Os-DMEDA) in the electronhistochemical study of nerve tissue. Proceedings of Histochemistry. pp. 519-520, 1972.
107) Haydée V. Castejón and Orlando J. Castejón: Application of Alcian Blue and Os- DMEDA in the electron histochemical study of cerebellar cortex. I. Alcian Blue staining. Symposium on Fine Structure of Cerebellum. Rev. Micr. Elec. Vol. 1, No. 2: 207-226. 1972.
108) Orlando J. Castejón and Haydée V. Castejón: Application of Alcian Blue and Os- DMEDA in the electron histochemical study of cerebellar cortex. II. Os-SMEDA staining. Symposium on Fine Structure of Cerebellum. Rev. Micr. Elec. Vol. 1, No. 2: 227-238. 1972.
109) Haydée V. Castejón, Orlando J. Castejón and Lourdes Salazar: Ultracytochemical demonstration of hyaluronidase-sensitive acidic glycosaminoglycans in cerebellar mossy fibres. Acta Científ. Venez. 24 (Sup. 1): 47, 1973.
110) Orlando J. Castejón, Haydée V. Castejón, María E. Viloria and Indalecio Rivero: Contribution of Ruthenium Chloride to the ultracytochemical study of cerebellar cortex. Proceedings XXXI Annual Meeting. Electron Microscopy Society of America. J. Arcceneau (Ed) New Orleans, USA. 1973, pp. 30-31.

111) María E. Vilora, Haydée V. Castejón, Orlando J. Castejón and Consuelo Valero: Different types of subsurface cisterns in mice and human central nervous systems. Proc. II Congreso Latinoamericano de Microscopia Electrónica Bello Horizonte. Brazil. pp. 134-135, 1974.

112) Castejón, Orlando J. and Castejón, Haydée V.: Application of GABOUL method to the ultracytochemical study of mouse blood-brain barrier. Proceedings Electron Microscopy Society of America. pp. 98-99, 1976.
113) Orlando J. Castejón and Haydée V. Castejón: The GABOUL method and its contribution to the ultracytochemical study of the cerebellar cortex. Electron Microscopy 1974. J. V. Sanders and D.J. Goodchild (Eds). Australian Academy of Science. Canberra, Australia. Vol. II, 1974, pp 328-329.
114) Orlando J. Castejón, Haydée V. Castejón, Consuelo Valero and María E. Viloria: Application of the GABOUL method to the ultracytochemical study of cerebellar capillaries. Acta Cientif. Venez. Vol. 25 (Sup. 1): 57-58, 1974.
115) Haydée V. Castejón, Orlando J. Castejón, María E. Viloria and Consuelo Valero: Ultracytochemical study of mouse cerebellar proteoglycans. Effect of methylation and enzymatic digestions. Proc. II Latin American Congress of Electron Microscopy. Bello Horizonte. Brazil: pp. 32-33, 1974.
116) Orlando J. Castejón and Haydée V. Castejón: Cytochemistry and ultrastructure of mouse and human cerebellar Golgi cells. Proc. II Congreso Latinoamericano de Microscopía Electrónica. Abstracts: pp. 34-35, 1974.
117) Consuelo Valero, Orlando J. Castejón, Haydée V. Castejón, María E. Viloria and José Ramón Guzmán: Electron microscopic study of perifocal edema associated to heman brain tumors. II Latin American Congress of Electron Microscopy. Bello Horizonte. Brazil. pp. 128-129,1974.
118) Viloria, María E.; Castejón, Haydée V. and Castejón, Orlando J.: Application of Alcian Blue to the submicroscopic study of capillary cells in human brain edema. Journal of Electron Microscopy, 3: 144-145, 1976.
119) Castejón, O.J. and Castejón, H.V.: Transmission and scanning electron microscopy and ultracytochemistry of vertebrate and human cerebellar cortex. In "Glial and Neuronal Cell Biology". Ed. Sergey Federoff, pp. 249-258, Alan R. Liss, Inc. New York, 1981.
120) Castejón, O.J.; Castejón, H.V.; Alvarado, M.E.; Montiel, N.J. and Espinoza, J.R.: The cerebellar stellate neurons. A freeze-fracture and ultrastructural study. Neuroscience Letters. Suppl. 22, 271-272, 1986.
121) Castejón, O.J. and Castejón, H.V.: Electron microscopy and glycosaminoglycan histochemistry of cerebellar stellate neurons. Scanning

Microscopy. 1, 681-693. 1987.
122) Perozo de R. S.; **Castejón, H. V.**, Falque L.: Anthropometric nutritional evaluation in a preschool population in marginal conditions. V Jornadas Científicas Facultad de Medicina. University of Zulia. 23-27 Sept. 1991. II National Congress of Nutrition. 1-4 April 1991. Maracaibo. Maracaibo, Venezuela. Published in Memorias del Congreso.
123) Perozo de R. S.; **Castejón, H. V.**, Falque L.: Anthropometric nutritional evaluation in children hospitalized in the Raul Leoni Hospital of Maracaibo and its correspondence with the basic pathology of admission. V Jornadas Científicas Facultad de Medicina. University of Zulia. 23-27 Sept. 1991. Maracaibo. Maracaibo, Venezuela . Published in Memorias del Jornadas.
124) Falque, L.; Andrade, E.; **Castejón, H. V.**: Anthropometric nutritional evaluation in a Nutritional Education and Recovery Service. IX Latin American Congress of Nutrition. 22-26 Sept. 1991. San Juan, Puerto Rico. . Published in Memorias del Congreso.
125) Méndez de G, N., Urrieta, R., Amaya de C.D., Molano, N., Zavala, M., Valero, C., Isambert, P., De la Cruz, C. and **Castejón, H. V.**: Relación de algunos indicadores antropométricos con el estado nutricional del zinc plasmático en niños desnutridos. X Latin American Congress of Nutrition. 13-18 Nov. 1994. Caracas. Caracas. Venezuela. Abstract in Archivos Latinomericanos de Nutrición 44(3): 145, 1994.
126) Venencia, I., Medrano de M., I., Méndez Gil N., **Castejón, H. V.**: Estudio de la talla baja en preescolares de la etnia guajira. VII Jornadas Científicas Fac. de Medicina. University of Zulia. 23-27 July, 1995. Maracaibo. Maracaibo. Venezuela. Invest. Clin. 36:74. 1995.
127) Andrade, E.; Molano. N.C.; **Castejón, H. V.**; Falque, L.M. and Pirela, L.: Nutritional recovery of children with the ambulatory administration of a food supplement (LACTOVISOY). III Jornadas Científicas de la Facultad de Medicina- Universidad del Zulia. September 21-25, 1987. Maracaibo. Maracaibo. Venezuela. Published in Memorias Jornadas.
128) Andrade, S.E.; Molano, N.C.; **Castejón, H. V.**; Falque, M.L. and Pirela, L.: Nutritional recovery of malnourished children with the ambulatory administration of a food supplement (LACTOVISOY). XXXVII Annual Convention of ASOVAC. 22-27 November 1987. Maracaibo. Maracaibo. Venezuela. Acta Científ. Venez. 38:216, 1987.
129) Castejón, H. V.: Functioning and importance of a Nutritional Education

and Recovery Service. Conference. Updating Workshop on Childhood Malnutrition. 18-22 March 1990. Maracaibo. Maracaibo. Venezuela.

130) Castejón H. V. Opportunities for action by nutritionists in health research programmes. Conference. II Jornadas Científicas del Colegio de Nutricionista de Venezuela. Sectional Zulia. "Dr. Francisco Solano Nava". Maracaibo 29 September - 4 October 1997.

131) Castejón, H.V. Monitoring the effectiveness of food programmes for marginalised pre-school and school children. Conference. IV Jornadas Científicas Colegio Nutricionistas - Dietistas de Venezuela seccional Zulia. "Yolanda Henriquez de Gonzalez". Maracaibo 22 - 23 July 1999.

132) Castejón, H.V. Evaluation and monitoring of nutritional intervention programmes. Conference at the Symposium "Nutritional intervention programmes for children in the State of Zulia". Current status and new alternatives. Coordinator Dr. Haydée V. Castejón. IX Scientific Conference of the Faculty of Medicine - LUZ. Maracaibo, 20 to 24 September 1999.

133) Mora de Suárez, A. ; **Castejón, H. V.** Soto, D.; Villarroel M.; Moreno, M.; Andrade, E.; Gil, N.M. Aggravation of child malnutrition detected in a screening consultation at the Chiquinquira Hospital in Maracaibo. V Jornadas Científicas Facultad de Medicina. University of Zulia. 23-27 Sept. 1991. Maracaibo. Maracaibo. Venezuela. Published in Memorias Jornadas.

134) **Castejón H. V.** Child Malnutrition. Its effects on the development of our children. Conference. VIII Jornadas Científicas Facultad de Medicina. University of Zulia. Maracaibo 20 -24 October 1997.

135) **Castejón H. V.** Some orientations on the prevention of malnutrition. Lecture at the Forum "Epidemiological profile of Zulia State". IV Jornadas Científicas XXX Aniversario de la Escuela de Nutrición y Dietética Facultad deMedicine - LUZ. Maracaibo, 28 June to 02 July 1998. Published in Libro Nutrición y Calidad de Vida. Ediluz (Ed) 155 - 157, 1998.

136) Gómez G; Ortega P; Alvarado N; Pérez M; **Castejón H.V.** Caloric and protein reserve in a marginal child population of Zulia State according to brachial measurements. IX Scientific Conference of the Faculty of Medicine - LUZ. Maracaibo, September 20-24, 1999. Clinical Research 40(Suppl 2): 149, 1999.

137) Gómez G; Ortega P; Alvarado N; Pérez M; Amaya D; Díaz ME; **Castejón H.V.** Anthropometric nutritional deficit in a child population of Zulia State with high food insecurity. IX Jornadas Científicas de la Facultad

de Medicina - LUZ. Maracaibo, 20-24 September 1999. Clinical Investigation 40(Suppl 2): 146 -147, 1999.

138) Molano NC, **Castejón HV**, Ortega P, Castejón OA. Evaluation of the admission and discharge conditions of malnourished children subject to comprehensive nutritional recovery in the nutritional education and recovery service (SERN) of the Chiquinquirá Hospital - National Institute of Nutrition (INN) in Maracaibo - Venezuela. XII Congress of the Latin American Society of Nutrition. Buenos Aires-Argentina, 12-16 November 2000. Book of Abstracts EN 2000.

139) Zambrano de Rodríguez, N.; Katiyar, V.; **Castejón, H. V.**; González, S. y Andrade, C.: Levels of urinary excretion of glucosaminoglycans and creatinine in malnourished children. XXXVI Annual Convention of ASOVAC. 16-21, November 1986. Valencia. Edo. Carabobo. Venezuela. Acta Científ. Venez. 37: 1986.

140) Amaya, D.; Katiyar, V.: **Castejón, H. V.** y Alvarado, M.E.: Glucosaminoglucan excretion values in urine of children with mental retardation. III Jornadas Científicas de la Facultad de Medicina-Universidad del Zulia. September 21-25, 1987. Maracaibo. Maracaibo. Venezuela. Published in Memorias Jornadas.

141) Katiyar V.N., **Castejón, H. V.**, Zambrano N., Urrieta J.; Alvarado, M.E. Identification and quantification of urinary glucosaminoglycans (GAG) in malnourished children from Maracaibo. XXXVII Annual ASOVAC Convention 22-27 Nov. 1988. Maracay. Venezuela. Acta. Sci. Venez. 39:152, 1988.

142) Zambrano, de R.N.; **Castejón, H. V.**; Falque, L.; Levels of urinary excretion of glucosaminoglycans in malnourished children. IX Latin American Congress of Nutrition. 22-26 Sept. 1991. San Juan, Puerto Rico. . Published in Memorias del Congreso.

143) Hudats, N., Higuera. N; **Castejón, H.V.**; Katiyar V., Méndez de Gil N.: Urinary protein excretion levels in normal and malnourished children in Maracaibo. XXXVII Annual Convention of ASOVAC. November 22-27, 1987. Maracaibo. Venezuela. Acta Científ. Venez. 38:215, 1987.

144) Marcucci, L.; Landaeta, M.; Ferrer, M.; Pirela, I.; Andrade, E.; Molano, N. and Castejón, H. V.: Intellectual development and social skills in children of low socioeconomic status. Their relationship with nutritional status. III Jornadas Científicas de la Facultad de Medicina, Universidad del Zulia.

September 21-25, 1987. Maracaibo. Maracaibo. Venezuela. Published in Memorias Jornadas.

145) Molano, N.C.; Ramírez, H. ; **Castejón, H.V.** ; Soto H.P. Andrade E. ; Boscán L. Plasma levels of immunoglobulins and serum complement in malnourished children in Maracaibo. XXXVII Annual Convention of ASOVAC. November 22-27, 1987. Maracaibo. Venezuela. Acta Científ. Venez. 38:198, 1987.

146) Molano, N., Urrieta, R., Méndez de Gil, N.; Zavala, M.; Valero, C.; Atencio, T.; **Castejón, H. V.**: Importance of plasma amino acid analysis in nutritional recovery. Pilot trial. VII Jornadas Científicas Fac. de Medicina. University of Zulia. 20-24, Sept. 1993. Maracaibo. Maracaibo, Venezuela . Published in Memorias Jornadas

147) Amaya, D., Méndez, N., Urrieta, R., Molano, N., Zavala, M., Valero, C., Ferrer, A., Moreno, L., Tineo, A., Castejón, H. V.: Plasma zinc levels in a marginal child population of Maracaibo. Pilot test. VII Jornadas Científicas Fac. de Medicina. University of Zulia. 20-24, Sept. 1993. Maracaibo. Venezuela.

148) Amaya de C.D., Urrieta, R., Méndez de G.N.; Molano, N., Valero, C., Ramos, M., Isambert, P., Atencio, T., Castejón, H. V., Niveles de Zinc plasmático en una población infantil marginal de Maracaibo. X Latin American Congress of Nutrition. Caracas 13-18 Nov., 1994. Abstract in Archivos Latinoamericanos de Nutrición 44(3): 33S, 1994. Caracas. Venezuela.

149) Ortega, P., Méndez de Gil, N., Medrano de M., I., Suárez, A., Venencia, I., Urrieta, J.R., Ramos, M., Valero, C., **Castejón, H. V.**: Plasma amino acids values in a marginal urban and middle class child population. VII Jornadas Científicas Fac. de Medicina. University of Zulia. 23-27 July, 1995. Maracaibo. Venezuela. Invest. Clin. 36:137-138. 1995.

150) Ortega, P., Méndez Gil, N., Medrano, I.; Atencio, T., Venencia, I., Urrieta, J.R., **Castejón, H. V.**: Plasma amino acid values in children with different degrees of malnutrition. VII Jornadas Científicas Fac. de Medicina. University of Zulia. July 23-27, 1995. Maracaibo. Maracaibo. Venezuela. Invest. Clin. 36:139. 1995.

151) Ortega, P., Méndez, N., Urrieta, J., Medrano I., Venencia, I., **Castejón, H. V.**: Utility of the non-essential/essential amino acid ratio (NEA/EA) indicator in the detection of early stages of protein-energy malnutrition.

XLVI Annual ASOVAC Convention. November 17-22, 1996. Barquisimeto. Barquisimeto. Venezuela. Acta Cient. Venez. Suppl. 1, 202, 1996.
152) Ortega, P., Méndez, N., Urrieta, J., Medrano, I., Venencia, I., **Castejón, H. V.**: Relation of the nutritional status of a child population with their plasma amino acid values. XLVI Annual ASOVAC Convention. November 17-22, 1996. Barquisimeto. Barquisimeto. Venezuela. Acta Cient. Venez. Suppl. 1, 202, 1996.
153) Castejón H. V., Ortega, P., Méndez, N., Urrieta, J. Plasma amino acid (AA) molar ratio as an index of early detection of protein malnutrition. VIII Jornadas Científicas Facultad de Medicina. University of Zulia. Maracaibo October 20 -24, 1997. Clinical Research 38(Suppl 1): 84, 1997.
154) Ortega, P., van Gelder, N.M., Castejón, HV., Gil, N.M., Urrieta, J.R. Socio- economic condition could affect plasma amino acid values in venezuelan children population. XI Congress of the Latin American Society of Nutrition "Dr. Abraham Horwizt". Guatemala City - Guatemala. November 9 - 15, 1997. Proceedings in Archivos Latinoamericanos de Nutrición (Suppl 1997).
155) Ortega, P., Castejón, HV., Méndez de Gil N., Medrano I., Urrieta, J.R. Imbalance of plasma valine as an early indicator of malnutrition. XLVII Annual Convention of AsoVAC. Valencia 16 - 21 November 1997. Acta Cientifica Venezolana (Suppl. 1): 156, 1997.

156) Amaya de C., D., Urrieta, R., Gil, N.M., Molano, M.C., Medrano, I., Castejón, H. V.: Plasma zinc values in a marginal child population of Maracaibo, Venezuela. Archivos Latinoamericanos de Nutrición, 47 (1): 2-28, 1997
157) Marquez, E., Castejón HV., Rangel, L., Medrano, I., Gómez, G., Hernández, D., Espina, D. PTU nutritional drink. Measurement of acceptance and tolerance. University Technological Park of Zulia. Maracaibo September 1997.
158) Marquez, E., León, N., Castejón HV., Rangel, L., Barboza, Y. Formulation and industrial trial of a long-life beverage with the company Sur del Lago. Parque Tecnológico Universitario del Zulia. Maracaibo December 1997.
159) Márquez E., Benítez, B., Méndez de G. N., Rangel L., Medrano I., Venencia I., Izquierdo P., Romero R., and Castejón H.V. Nutritional characteristics of a biscuit formulated with bovine blood plasma as the main

protein source. Archivos Latinoamericanos de Nutricion 48 (3): 250 - 255, 1998.

160) Rangel, L., León, N., Castejón, HV. Marquez, E., Benitez, B., Barboza, Y. Formulation and chemical nutritional evaluation of a sterilised infant food, based on soy isolate, whey and milk, for social nutritional programmes. IX Jornadas Científicas de la Facultad de Medicina - LUZ. Maracaibo, 20-24 September 1999. Clinical Research 40(Suppl 2): 147 - 148, 1999.

161) Ortega, P., van Gelder, N.M., Castejón, HV., Gil, N.M., Urrieta, J.R. Plasma amino acids as potential markers of child malnutrition. Conference. Winner of the "Dr. Francisco Solano Nava" award. Edition 1998. IV Scientific Conference XXX Anniversary of the School of Nutrition and Dietetics Faculty of Medicine - LUZ. Maracaibo, June 28th to July 2nd, 1998.

162) Ortega, P., Castejón, H.V., Méndez de Gil, N., Medrano, I., Venencia, I., Urrieta, J. Comparative study of plasma amino acid values between Goajira and non-Goajira pre-schoolers in Maracaibo. Pilot test. XLVIII Annual Convention of AsoVAC - 1998. Maracaibo, 9 to 13 November 1998.

163) Ortega, P., van Gelder, N.M., Castejón, HV, Gil, N.M., Urrieta, J.R. Imbalance of individual plasma amino acids relative to valine and taurine as potential markers of childhood malnutrition. Nutritional Neuroscience 2:163 -173, 1999.

164) Ortega, P., Gómez, G., Alvarado, N., Pérez, M., León de Yordi, L., Castejón, H.V. Haematological values in marginal pre-schoolers, beneficiaries or not of a complementary nutritional programme. IX Jornadas Científicas de la Facultad de Medicina - LUZ. Maracaibo, 20-24 September 1999. Clinical Research 40 (Suppl 2) : 146,1999.

165) Ortega, P., Gómez, G., Díaz, M.E., Amaya, D., Castejón, H.V. Iron deficiency anemia and sub-clinical deficiency of vitamin A in a marginal pre-school population of Zulia State, Venezuela. IL Annual Convention of AsoVAC - 1999. Maracay, 14-19 November 1999. Acta Científica Venezolana, 50, Suppl. 2, p. 231, 1999.

166) Integral nutritional study and analysis of the nutritional effectiveness of the food programme applied to pre-school children attending the Santa Ana Foundation canteen, Maracaibo Municipality, Zulia State. Responsible: Dr. Pablo Ortega, Lic. Gisela Gómez. Advisor: Dr. Haydée V. Castejón. May

1999.

167) Integral nutritional study of children attending the "Romulo Gallegos I" pre-school, Maracaibo Municipality, Zulia State. Responsible: Dr. Pablo Ortega, Lic. Gisela Gómez. Advisor: Dr. Haydée V. Castejón. May 1999

168) Díaz, M.E., Amaya, D., Ortega, P., Gómez, G., Alvarado, N., Ramos, M., Castejón,

H.V. Nutritional status of vitamin A in a marginal pre-school population of Zulia State by means of conjunctival impression cytology study. IX Scientific Conference of the Faculty of Medicine - LUZ. Maracaibo, September 20-24, 1999. Clinical Research 40(Suppl 2) : 148 - 149, 1999.

169) Amaya, D. , Diaz, ME., Gómez, G.,Ortega, P., Ramos, M. , Castejón, HV. Prevalence of sub-clinic vitamin A deficiency and malnutrition in preschool children of Zulia State, Venezuela. IL AsoVAC Annual Convention - 1999. Maracay, 14-19 November 1999. Acta Científica Venezolana, 50, Suppl. 2, 1999.

170) Ortega P, Castejón HV, Amaya D, Gómez G, Urrieta JR, Díaz ME. Conditioning risk factors for subclinical vitamin A deficiency in a paediatric population. Maracaibo-Venezuela. XII Congress of the Latin American Society of Nutrition. Buenos Aires-Argentina, 12-16 November 2000. Book of Abstracts EN 224, 2000.

171) Amaya D, Castejón HV, Ortega P, Gómez G, Urrieta JR, Díaz ME. Nutritional status of vitamin A in a marginalized infant population of Maracaibo, Zulia State - Venezuela. XII Congress of the Latin American Society of Nutrition. Buenos Aires-Argentina, 12-16 November 2000. Book of Abstracts EN 66, 2000.

172) Ortega P, Castejón HV, Amaya D, Urrieta JR, Gómez G, Díaz M, Ramos M and Lobo P. Is anaemia a good predictor of vitamin A deficiency (VAD) or is VAD a good predictor of anaemia? L Annual Convention of AsoVAC. Caracas, November 19-24, 2000. Acta Cient. Venez. 51. Suppl 2: 157, 2000.

173) Amaya D, Castejón HV, Ortega P, Urrieta JR, Gómez G, Lobo P, Díaz M. Serum vitamin A values in a marginalized child population in the Maracaibo area, Venezuela. L Annual Convention of AsoVAC. Caracas, November 19-24, 2000. Acta Cient. Venez. 51. Suppl 2: 157, 2000.

174) Castejón HV, Ortega P, Amaya D, Urrieta JR, Gómez G, Díaz M, Ramos

M and Lobo P. Conjunctival impression cytology (CIC) versus serum retinol to detect subclinical vitamin A deficiency in marginalized children in Maracaibo. L Annual Convention of AsoVAC. Caracas, November 19-24, 2000. Acta Cient. Venez. 51. Suppl 2: 158, 2000.

175) **Castejón OJ, Apkarian RP, Castejón HV. Field emission scanning electron microscopy and** freeze-fracture transmission electron microscopy of mouse cerebellar synaptic contacts. Annual Meeting Society for Neuroscience. New Orleans. NEW ORLEANS. November, 4-11, 2000.

176) **Castejón OJ, Apkarian RP, Castejón HV. Field emission scanning electron microscopy and** freeze-fracture transmission electron microscopy of mouse cerebellar synaptic contacts. Annual Meeting Society for Neuroscience. New Orleans. NEW ORLEANS. November, 4-11, 2000.

177) Rangel L., León N., Castejón H.V. Barboza Y., Zarraga I., Gómez G., Medrano I., Márquez E., Formulation and chemical-nutritional evaluation of a foodstuff. sterilised soy isolate, whey and milk for school children. Anales Venezolanos de Nutricion 13: 181 - 187, 2000.

178) Castejón HV, Amaya D, Ortega P, Gómez G, Urrieta JR y Lobo P. Anthropometric nutritional status and vitamin A deficiency in children from Zulia State. X Jornadas Científicas de la Facultad de Medicina. Maracaibo, 29 October to 2 November 2001. Clinical Research 42 (Suppl. 2): 129 - 130, 2001.

179) Ortega P., Castejón HV., Argotte M., Bohórquez L., Gómez G., Urrieta JR. Gestational variations in plasma amino acid concentration in healthy adolescents from Maracaibo, Venezuela. LI Annual Convention of AsoVAC. San Cristobal, November 18-23, 2001. Acta Cient. Venez. 52. Suppl 3: 192, 2001.

180) Ortega P., Castejón HV., Argotte M., Bohórquez L., Gómez G., Urrieta JR. Plasma amino acid profile in a population of adolescents with adequate nutrition in Maracaibo, Venezuela. LI Annual Convention of AsoVAC. San Cristobal, November 18-23, 2001. Acta Cient. Venez. 52. Suppl 3: 194, 2001.

181) Ortega P, Castejón HV, Gómez G, Castejón C, Vargas V, Prevalence of anaemia in pregnant women at term in Maracaibo. Effects on the newborn X Jornadas Científicas de la Facultad de Medicina. Maracaibo, 29 October to 2 November 2001. Clinical Research 42 (Suppl. 2): 88, 2001.

182) Ortega P, Castejón HV, Gómez G, Castejón C, Vargas V. Parity and

maternal anaemia in a sample of pregnant women in Maracaibo. Effects on the neonate. X Jornadas Científicas de la Facultad de Medicina. Maracaibo, 29 October to 2 November 2001. Clinical Research 42 (Suppl. 2): 88 - 89, 2001.

183) Bohórquez L, Gómez G, Mejías L, Ortega P, Chirinos M, Castejón HV. Nutritional evaluation of female adolescents in Maracaibo. LIII Annual Convention of AsoVAC. Maracaibo, 25-29 November 2003. Castejón HV, Ortega P, Díaz ME, Amaya D, Gómez G, Ramos M, Alvarado ME, Urrieta JR. Prevalence of subclinical vitamin A deficiency and malnutrition in marginal children in Maracaibo - Venezuela. Arch Latinoamer Nutr 51, 25 - 32, 2001.

184) Gómez G, Ortega P, Urrieta JR, Castejón HV. Percentage of adequacy of daily vitamin A intake in a marginal child population in Zulia State. Relationship with vitamin A deficiency. X Jornadas Científicas de la Facultad de Medicina. Maracaibo, October 29th to November 2nd, 2001. Clinical Research 42 (Suppl. 2): 145, 2001.

185) Amaya D, Castejón HV, Ortega P, Gómez G, Urrieta JR y Lobo P. Hypovitaminosis A in a sample of marginal children from Zulia State. Predisposing factors. X Jornadas Científicas de la Facultad de Medicina. Maracaibo, October 29th to November 2nd, 2001. Clinical Research 42 (Suppl. 2): 142, 2001.

186) Castejon HV. Vitamin A nutritional supplementation programme. Present and future. Conference. Symposium Update in the management of micronutrient deficiencies. X Jornadas Cientificas, Faculty of Medicine, University of Zulia. Maracaibo, 2 November 2001.

187) Castejon HV. Suggestion for the application of food programmes for pre-school and marginalised school children. Conference. Round Table, Malnutrition and Experiences in Education and Nutritional Recovery Programmes. XLVIII Annual Assembly and Scientific Conference of the Venezuelan Society of Public Health. Maracaibo, 30 November 2001

188) Ortega P., Castejón HV., Gómez G., Ocando M., Molano N. Prevalence of anaemia and iron deficiency in pre-school children in Maracaibo, Venezuela. LII Annual Convention of AsoVAC. Barquisimeto, November 17-22, 2002. Acta Cient. Venez. 53. Suppl 1: 29, 2002.

189) Amaya-Castellano D. Viloria Castejon H., Ortega P., Gomez G., Urrieta JR. Lobo P., Estevez J. Vitamin A deficiency and anthropometric

nutritional status in marginal urban and rural children in Zulia State, Venezuela. Clinical Research, 43:89-105, 2002.

190) Castejón HV., Castejón JA., Ortega P., Amaya D., Gómez G., Leal J., Molano N. Efficacy of a nutritional supplement in the correction of subclinical vitamin A deficiency in pre-school children in Maracaibo, Venezuela. LII Annual Convention of AsoVAC. Barquisimeto, November 17-22, 2002. Acta Cient. Venez. 53. Suppl 1: 28, 2002

191) Leal J, Castejón HV, Romero T, Ortega P, Gómez G. Decreased serum concentration of interleukin 10 in preschoolers with subclinical vitamin A deficiency. XIII Latin American Congress of Nutrition "Nutrition for life". Acapulco City - Mexico, 09-13 November 2000. Latin American Archives of Nutrition. 2003.

192) Castejón HV, Ortega P, Amaya D, Gómez G, Leal J. Prevalence of anaemia, vitamin A deficiency and height and weight deficits in children from marginal communities of Maracaibo, Venezuela. LIII Annual Convention of AsoVAC. Maracaibo, 25-29 November 2003.

193) Ortega P, Castejón HV, Amaya D, Gómez G, Leal J. Anthropometric profile and erythrocyte indices in preschoolers with anemia and vitamin A deficiency. LIII Annual Convention of AsoVAC. Maracaibo, 25-29 November 2003.

194) Leal J, Rodríguez M, Castejón HV, Ortega P, Gómez G, Amaya D. Anaemia in eutrophic children parasitized by giardia lamblia. LIII Annual Convention of AsoVAC. Maracaibo, 25-29 November 2003.

195) Leal J, Rodríguez M, Castejón HV, Ortega P, Gómez G, Amaya D. Anaemia and intestinal parasitosis in children from Maracaibo-Venezuela. LIII Annual Convention of the AsoVAC. Maracaibo, 25-29 November 2003.

196) Gómez G, Leal J, Ortega P, Amaya D, Castejón HV. Vitamin A deficiency in children from marginal communities of Maracaibo. Dietary evaluation. LIII Annual Convention of AsoVAC. Maracaibo, 25-29 November 2003.

197) Mejía L, Gómez G, Bohórquez L, Ortega P, Leal J, Castejón HV. Dietary evaluation of pregnant adolescents in Maracaibo Venezuela. LIII Annual Convention of AsoVAC. Maracaibo, 25-29 November 2003.

198) Ortega P., Castejón HV., Argotte M., Gómez G., Bohorquez L., Urrieta JR. Plasma amino acid profile in healthy pregnant adolescents from Maracaibo, Venezuela. Arch Latinoamer Nutr. 53 (2): 157-164.2003.

199) Ortega P, Castejón HV, Leal J, Mejía L, Chirinos N. Anaemia and iron deficiency in pregnant adolescents in Maracaibo - Venezuela. XIII Congress of the Latin American Society of Nutrition. Acapulco City - Mexico, November 09-13, 2000. Latin American Archives of Nutrition. 2003.

200) Castejón HV, Ortega P, Amaya D, Gómez G, Leal J. Co-existence of anemia, vitamin A deficiency and growth retardation among children 24 - 84 months old in Maracaibo, Venezuela. Nutritional Neuroscience. 7(2): 113-119. 2004

201) Leal J, Castejón HV, Romero T, Ortega P, Gómez G, Amaya D, Estévez J. Serum cytokine values in children with vitamin A deficiency disorders. Invest. Clin. 45(3): 243 - 256. 2004.

202) Leal J, Castejón HV, Romero T, Ortega P, Gómez G, Amaya D. Serum values of interleukin 10 appear diminished in children with vitamin A deficiency disorders. XXII IVACG Meeting Vitamin A and The Common agenda for micronutrients. Lima, Peru, 15-17 November 2004.

203) Castejón HV, Ortega P, Amaya D, Gómez G, Leal J. Co-existence of anaemia, vitamin a deficiency and growth retardation among children 24-84 months old in Maracaibo, Venezuela. XXII IVACG Meeting Vitamin A and The common Agenda for micronutrients. Lima, Peru, 15-17 November 2004.

More than a hundred publications, often in collaboration with her husband Dr. Orlando Castejón. Orlando Castejón, enabled her to continue her original publications in Acta Histochemica (Germany), Journal of Histochemistry and Cytochemistry (USA), Histochemie (France), Cell and Molecular Biology (Paris), Journal Submicroscopic Cytology and Pathology (Italy), Revista de Microscopía Electronica (Venezuela), Biocell (Argentina), Journal of Neuroscience Research (USA, International Journal of Developmental Neuroscience (England), Neuroscience Letters (USA), Scanning Microscopy (USA), Scanning (USA) Histology and Histopathology (Spain), Revista Española de Neurología (Madrid), Trabajos del Instituto Cajal (Madrid), and Brain Injury (USA).In the 1990s, he began to apply his fundamental research to the study of child malnutrition, when he discovered that malnourished children did not have the protein levels to combine with proteoglycans. With an interdisciplinary group of more than twenty professionals, including researchers, paediatricians, nutritionists and psychologists, he founded the Nutrition Service of the Chiquinquirá Hospital in Maracaibo. Here he carries out clinical research on malnourished children in hospital and in consultation. Subsequently, he also organised the Laboratory of Child Malnutrition at the Hospital de Especialidades Pediátricas de Maracaibo, where he worked with his most recent disciples, Drs. Pablo Ortega and Jorimar Leal. Both institutions are attached to the Institute of Biological Research. This new research programme has resulted in notable publications, highly appreciated by the World Health Organisation in Geneva, and published in journals such as Nutritional Neuroscience (USA), Anales Venezolanos de Nutrición and Archivos Latinoamericanos de Nutrición e Investigación Clínica (Venezuela).During his academic career he received numerous distinctions and awards, among them: Orden al Mérito Universitario Dr Jesús Enrique Losada, Orden Andrés Bello, Distinción a la Mujer Creativa del Zulia, Premio Dr Francisco Solano Nava, Premio Honor al Mérito Científico de Fundacite Zulia, Profesor Meritorio del CONABA, and Investigador Nivel III de la Fundación Programa de Promoción del Investigador del Ministerio de Ciencia y Tecnología de Venezuela. By decision of the Council of the Faculty of Medicine and the University Council of LUZ, her name together with that of her husband were designated to honour the name of the Institute of Biological Research of the Faculty of Medicine of LUZ. At the time of her death, Dr Castejón was being nominated for the UNESCO Loreal Prize for Women in Science in Paris.He actively participated in the foundation and development of scientific societies in Venezuela and Latin America: Asociación Venezolana para el Avance de la Ciencia. Zuliano Chapter (1967), Venezuelan and Latin American Societies of Electron Microscopy (1972), Venezuelan Society of Histochemistry and Cytochemistry (1982), Iberoamerican Federation of Histochemistry and Cytochemistry (1989-1992), Venezuelan Society of Neurosciences, as well as actively participating in the Organising Commission of the Congresses of these Societies, of which he was President. He also participated in the development and promotion of the technical commissions of the scientific policy bodies in Venezuela, such as El Conicit (Caracas), (1973-1979), Consejo de Desarrollo Científico y Humanístico de LUZ (1988-1990), Fundacite Zulia, Consejo de la Facultad y Consejo Técnico de Postgrado de la Facultad de Medicina de LUZ (1984-1992). She has been a lecturer in the area of postgraduate studies and research, acting as a tutor for more than 27 undergraduate and postgraduate theses. She founded a true school of research through the formation of a group of more than forty researchers and associated professionals for the Venezuelan Universities. With her death, the Venezuelan and international scientific community loses one of its most notable leaders and one of its most outstanding human values. Dr. Haydée Viloria de Castejón is an example for young Latin American scholars, a woman of universal science and an exceptional spiritual and religious figure.

CHAPTER XII

PROFILE OF DR. HAYDEE VILORIA DE CASTEJÓN

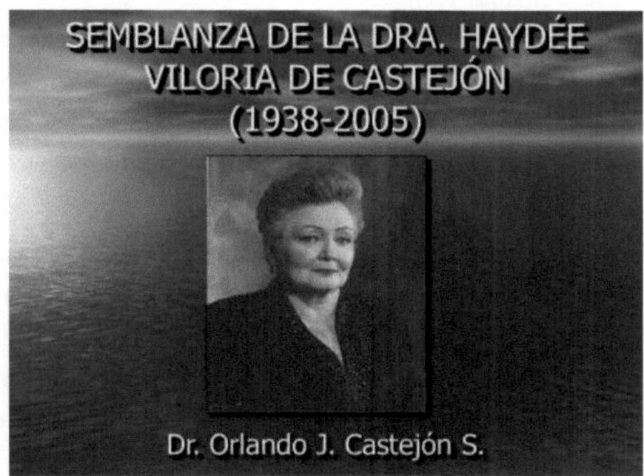

Orlando J. Castejón, Director of the Clinical Neurosciences Institute, Hogar Clínica San Rafael de Maracaibo. Castejón Foundation. Institute of Biological Research Drs Orlando J, Castejón and Haydee Viloria de Castejón. Faculty of Medicine, University of Zulia. ocastejo81@gmail.com

Dr. Haydée Viloria de Castejón was born in Maracaibo, Venezuela, on February 2, 1938, to Mr. Luis Enrique Viloria and Mrs. Julia Ocando de Viloria. From an early age she received her primary and secondary education at the Colegio del Pilar, where she obtained her sixth grade certificate and her bachelor's degree in Biological Sciences (1945-1956).

His time at the Colegio del Pilar, a Catholic school par excellence, imbued him with a strong religious spirit which he would express on a daily basis in his family environment, in his social environment and in his future scientific activity for the rest of his life. During his first year of medical school, he met Orlando Castejón Sandoval, at that time a trainer in the Department of Human Anatomy, under the direction of Dr. Julio Cesar García. From that meeting in the corridors of the School of Medicine came the friendship and love that would unite them for half a century in love and science.In 1957, she was appointed Trainer of the Department of Histology and Embryology, when she was in her second year of Medicine, receiving practical training and teaching under the direction of Professors Romer Irragorry, Romer Homez and Franz Wenger. In 1958, he joined the group of students who, under the direction of Dr. Américo Negrette, founded the Clinical Research Centre at the School of Medicine, under the direction of Dr. Vinicio Arrieta. The following students, among others, were part of that group: Elena and Slavia Ryder, Herman Serrano, Orlando Castejón and Dora Freites. On 18 August 1960, as a student in her fifth year of Medicine, she married Br. Orlando Castejón Sandoval, a student in his sixth year of Medicine. On 27 July 1962, he received his degree in Surgery from Dr. Antonio Borjas Romero, the Eternal Rector of LUZ.In 1962 he became a Graduate Student at the Instituto Venezolano de Investigaciones Científicas (IVIC), working under the direction of Dr. Luis Carbonell, Head of the Department of Histochemistry and Experimental Pathology, and current President of the Venezuelan Academy of Medicine. In 1964, she completed her postgraduate studies at the University of California, Los Angeles (UCLA), in the Department of Zoology, under the direction of Professor Fritiof Sjöstrand, and at the Brain Research Institute of the same University, under the direction of Dr. Jan Brown. In 1965, she became a founding member of the Clinical Research Centre of the Faculty of Medicine of LUZ, now the Clinical Research Institute, under the direction of Dr. Americo Negrette. There she founded the Histochemistry and Cytochemistry Section, and began her studies on histochemistry under the optical microscope. and electronics of proteoglycans in the vertebrate central nervous system.From 1965 to 1972 she worked with her husband Dr. Orlando Castejón on the electron microscopic identification of proteoglycans in mouse nerve cells. During this period she published in Acta Histochemica (Germany). Histochemie (France), Journal of Histochemistry and Cytochemistry (USA), and Revista de Microscopía Electrónica (Venezuela).In 1971, together with her husband, she founded the Biological Research Unit of the Faculty of Medicine, now the Institute of Biological Research, to promote the development of biomedical research in the basic medical sciences. At this Institution she continued her research and designed the GABOUL Method for the characterisation of proteoglycans in nerve cells. These findings, made in the period 1972-1990, allowed him to further study these macromolecules in all vertebrate species, including man. She then went on to explore the presence of these compounds during embryological development, with the collaboration of Dr. María Elena Viloria, Dr. Clarisa Faría, Dr. María Elena González, as well as

numerous students and professors from the Faculty of Medicine, Sciences and Humanities. Dr. Castejón thus emerged as one of the pioneers in her field of research at an international level, widely recognised for her systematic, honest, highly critical and rigorous work. She was characterised by her rational use of the scientific method and its applications, intuitively following the postulates of the philosophy of science. She admired Don Santiago Ramón y Cajal, the illustrious Spanish neurohistologist, founder of neurosciences and Nobel Prize for Medicine, Madame Curie, of whom she always kept a beautiful photo in her laboratory, and Claude Bernard, the founder of Experimental Medicine in France. Born in Maracaibo, her spirit was essentially European.More than a hundred publications, often in collaboration with her husband Dr. Orlando Castejón, allowed her to continue her original publications in Acta Histochemica (Germany), Journal of Histochemistry and Cytochemistry (USA), Histochemie (France), Cell and Molecular Biology (USA), and in the journal "Cell and Molecular Biology" (France). (Paris), Journal Submicroscopic Cytology and Pathology (Italy), Revista de Microscopía Electronica (Venezuela), Biocell (Argentina), Journal of Neuroscience Research (USA), International Journal of Developmental Neuroscience (England), Neuroscience Letters (USA), Scanning Microscopy (USA), Scanning (USA) Histology and Histopathology (Spain), Revista Española de Neurología (Madrid), Trabajos del Instituto Cajal (Madrid), and Brain Injury (USA).In the 1990s, he began to apply his fundamental research to the study of child malnutrition, when he discovered that malnourished children did not have the protein levels to combine with proteoglycans. With an interdisciplinary group of more than twenty professionals, including researchers, paediatricians, nutritionists and psychologists, he founded the Nutrition Service of the Chiquinquirá Hospital in Maracaibo, where he carried out clinical research on malnourished children in hospital and in consultation. Subsequently, he also organised the Laboratory of Child Malnutrition at the Hospital de Especialidades Pediátricas de Maracaibo, where he worked with his most recent disciples, Drs. Pablo Ortega and Jorimar Leal. Both institutions are attached to the Instituto de Investigaciones Biológicas. This new research programme has resulted in notable publications, highly appreciated by the World Health Organisation in Geneva, and published in journals such as Nutritional Neuroscience (USA), Anales Venezolanos de Nutrición and Archivos Latinoamericanos de Nutrición e Investigación Clínica (Venezuela).During his academic career he received numerous distinctions and

awards, among them: Orden al Mérito Universitario Dr Jesús Enrique Losada, Orden Andrés Bello, Distinción a la Mujer Creativa del Zulia, Premio Dr Francisco Solano Nava, Premio Honor al Mérito Científico de Fundacite Zulia, Profesor Meritorio del CONABA, and Investigador Nivel III de la Fundación Programa de Promoción del Investigador del Ministerio de Ciencia y Tecnología de Venezuela.By decision of the Council of the Faculty of Medicine and the University Council of LUZ, her name together with that of her husband were designated to honour the name of the Institute of Biological Research of the Faculty of Medicine. of LUZ. At the time of her death, Dr Castejón was being nominated for the UNESCO Loreal Prize for Women in Science in Paris.He actively participated in the foundation and development of scientific societies in Venezuela and Latin America: Asociación Venezolana para el Avance de la Ciencia. Zuliano Chapter (1967), Venezuelan and Latin American Societies of Electron Microscopy (1972), Venezuelan Society of Histochemistry and Cytochemistry (1982), Iberoamerican Federation of Histochemistry and Cytochemistry (1989-1992), Venezuelan Society of Neurosciences, as well as actively participating in the Organising Commission of the Congresses of these Societies, of which he was President. He also participated in the development and promotion of the technical commissions of the scientific policy bodies in Venezuela, such as El Conicit (Caracas), (1973-1979), Consejo de Desarrollo Científico y Humanístico de LUZ (1988-1990), Fundacite Zulia, Consejo de la Facultad y Consejo Técnico de Postgrado de la Facultad de Medicina de LUZ (1984-1992).She has been a lecturer in the area of postgraduate studies and research, acting as a tutor for more than 27 undergraduate and postgraduate theses. She founded a true school of research through the formation of a group of more than forty researchers and associated professionals for the Venezuelan Universities. With his death, the Venezuelan and international scientific community loses one of its most notable leaders and one of its most outstanding human values. Dr Haydée Viloria de Castejón is an example for young Latin American scholars, a woman of universal science and an exceptional spiritual and religious figure.

MIX
Papier aus verantwortungsvollen Quellen
Paper from responsible sources
FSC® C105338

Printed by Books on Demand GmbH, Norderstedt / Germany